Core Topics in Operating Department Practice

Leadership and Management

Core Topics in **Operating Department Practice**

Leadership and Management

Edited by

Brian Smith

Paul Rawling

Paul Wicker

Chris Jones

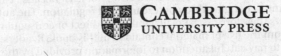

CAMBRIDGE
UNIVERSITY PRESS

University Printing House, Cambridge CB2 8BS, United Kingdom

One Liberty Plaza, 20th Floor, New York, NY 10006, USA

477 Williamstown Road, Port Melbourne, VIC 3207, Australia

314-321, 3rd Floor, Plot 3, Splendor Forum, Jasola District Centre, New Delhi - 110025, India

79 Anson Road, #06-04/06, Singapore 079906

Cambridge University Press is part of the University of Cambridge.

It furthers the University's mission by disseminating knowledge in the pursuit of education, learning and research at the highest international levels of excellence.

www.cambridge.org
Information on this title: www.cambridge.org/9780521717045

First published 2010

A catalogue record for this publication is available from the British Library

Library of Congress Cataloging in Publication data
Core topics in operating department practice : leadership and management / [edited by] Brian Smith . . . [et al.].
     p.   cm.
   ISBN 978-0-521-71704-5 (pbk.)
  1.   Health services administration. I.   Smith, Brian, 1965 Nov. 15– II.   Title.
   RA971.C737 2010
   362.1068–dc22

2009030227

ISBN 978-0-521-71704-5 Paperback

Additional resources for this publication at www.cambridge.org/delange

Cambridge University Press has no responsibility for the persistence or accuracy of URLs for external or third-party internet websites referred to in this publication, and does not guarantee that any content on such websites is, or will remain, accurate or appropriate.

....

Contents

Contributors

Lee Bennett
Alderhey Children's NHS Foundation Trust
Alderhey Hospital
Liverpool, UK

Claire Campbell
NHS North Lancashire
Lancaster, UK

Ian Cumming
NHS North Lancashire
Lancaster, UK

Rita J Hehir
Edge Hill University
Ormskirk
Lancashire, UK

Jean Hinton
Edge Hill University
Ormskirk
Lancashire, UK

Anne Jones
Edge Hill University
Ormskirk
Lancashire, UK

Chris Jones
Edge Hill University
Ormskirk
Lancashire, UK

Jill MacKeen
Faculty of Health
ODP Education
Ormskirk
Lancashire, UK

Sherran Milton
Association for Perioperative Practice
Harrogate
North Yorkshire, UK

Charlotte Moen
Edge Hill University
Ormskirk
Lancashire, UK

Peter Norman
NHS Purchasing and Supply Agency
Chester, UK

Joy O'Neill
Edge Hill University
Ormskirk
Lancashire, UK

Trish Prescott
Edge Hill University
Ormskirk
Lancashire, UK

Paul Rawling
Edge Hill University
Ormskirk
Lancashire, UK

Judith Roberts
Edge Hill University
Ormskirk
Lancashire, UK

Brian Smith
Edge Hill University
Ormskirk
Lancashire, UK

Julie Smith
St Helens & Knowsley Hospital Trust
Whiston Hospital
Prescot
Merseyside, UK

Lorraine Thomas
Aintree University Hospitals NHS Foundation Trust
University Hospital Aintree
Liverpool, UK

Paul Wicker
Edge Hill University
Ormskirk
Lancashire, UK

Foreword

So, what makes a good leader? Are leaders made or born? Is management a science or an art? The attributes of good leaders and managers are inextricably linked and have been defined as integrity, business understanding, consistency, ability to admit to mistakes, ability to listen and decisiveness. These are attributes that, I am sure, we would all aspire to emulate. I would also add 'patience' to this list, as good work does not happen overnight. A familiar comment by Eisenhower is a particular favourite of mine: 'leadership is the art of getting someone else to do something you want done because he wants to do it'.

Good leadership and management are synonymous with change, something we are all familiar with in healthcare. During the last 10 years, healthcare has moved forward at breakneck speed. This has put healthcare professionals in expanding circles of influence. We are now aware of how our actions are governed, or managed, on both a micro- and a macrolevel. This self-awareness of our professional personae has encouraged us to lead, although we might not be aware that we are leaders. Whether it is leading patients through difficult times, leading students on their path to professional fulfilment or leading our teams through challenging days, we as professionals must lead through an ever-changing landscape within healthcare.

So how do we prepare for these changes? Education and training is the core of our delivery of an excellent service to our patients. How we learn and what we learn has also changed. Technological advances and issues of professional boundaries and competence have impacted on the perioperative environment in such a way as to splinter the very existence of what was considered the norm. New technologies have impacted on delivery of, and teaching in, healthcare. This has resulted in improving communication and technological advances in treatment that, ultimately, are accelerating the patient's perioperative journey. These advances have also resulted in professional boundaries being pushed to their limits, with blurring of roles and responsibilities of members within the multidisciplinary healthcare team.

Questions of professionalism linked to competency and regulation have been emphasized to the public and highlighted by the media in cases such as those of Harold Shipman and Beverly Allitt (Department of Health 2006a). The media attention has also had adverse effects on public confidence in healthcare and has emphasized the requirement for competent practitioners to be transparent about the regulatory mechanisms that govern them (Department of Health 2006b). This has made both the medical profession and the public aware of the need for change within the regulatory mechanisms that govern our contemporary healthcare workers (Hewitt 2007). The realism of today's healthcare is that the lines of professional boundaries have blurred, with many qualified and unqualified practitioners now performing extended roles that 10 years ago were not even in existence (Department of Health 2007). Many of these roles were deemed necessary to fill the skills' gap created by the working time directive (Income Data Services 2007) and the reduction in doctors' working hours (Cass *et al.* 2003). This created new opportunities for a multitude of extended roles for existing healthcare professionals, such as nurses and operating department practitioners, and also for the creation of new professions within the perioperative arena, such as surgical care practitioners and anaesthetic practitioners.

Other issues that have impacted on the contemporary healthcare workforce include comprehensive changes in pay with the introduction of the *Agenda for Change,* which is inextricably linked to the *NHS Knowledge and Skills Framework* (KSF) (Department of Health 2004). The NHS KSF and its associated development review process are designed to define the knowledge and skills required by NHS staff to function within their designated role, with the intention that the 'KSF lies at the heart of the career progression strand of the Agenda for Change'.

So again I will ask the question, what makes a good leader? Is the answer the charisma of leaders and their ability to communicate a vision (Tomey 1993)? Maybe, as all great leaders and managers have charisma. However, good leadership and management go beyond charisma. Perhaps I can sum it up by saying, I don't know what makes a good leader; but I know when I've been led.

Sherran Milton

REFERENCES

Cass, H. D., Smith, I., Unthank, C., Starling, C. & Collins, J. (2003). Improving compliance with requirements on junior doctors' hours. *British Medical Journal*, **327**, 270–273.

Department of Health (2004). *The NHS Knowledge and Skills Framework (NHS KSF) and the Development Review Process*. London: The Stationery Office.

Department of Health (2006a). *Good Doctors, Safer Patients*. London: The Stationery Office.

Department of Health (2006b). *The Regulation of the Non-medical Healthcare Professions*. London: The Stationery Office.

Department of Health (2007). *NHS Modernisation Agency Collaboration Tools*. London: The Stationery Office.

Hewitt, P. (2007). *Trust, Assurance and Safety: The Regulation of Health Professionals in the 21st Century*. London: The Stationery Office.

Income Data Services (2007). *European Working Time Directive*. London: Income Data Services; http://www.incomesdata.co.uk/information/worktimedirective.htm (accessed 21 July 2009).

Tomey, A. M. (1993). *Transformational Leadership in Nursing*. London: Mosby.

Preface

This is the second book in the *Core Topics in Operating Department Practice* series. Following the overwhelming success of the first book, *Anaesthesia and Critical Care*, we offer this leadership and managerial text as another reference point for practising and studying perioperative practitioners.

The motivation in compiling this book was the observation that, despite the immense complexity of managing a modern operating theatre suite, books aimed at addressing issues for theatre managers were few in number. This remarkable fact is hard to explain given that sound management and effective leadership are regarded as key factors in health service modernization. Indeed, the need for strong and effective leadership is one of the few points on which operating department practitioners, nurses, medical staff, politicians and patients can agree upon in developing services in the new century.

Taking the same approach as our first book, colleagues from a variety of backgrounds have kindly given up their time to share their expertise in numerous fields, such as corporate governance, the development of advanced roles, the management of cultural diversity in the perioperative environment and the influence of organizational culture in the day-to-day life of a theatre suite. Each chapter explores the topic in a clear authoritative style, giving personal experiences to illustrate how some issues could be overcome and could reshape the patient's experience.

We hope that each chapter will enable the reader to develop skills that will be useful in setting into theoretical context the demands of everyday practice. We hope that chapters such as 'Leadership in Perioperative Settings: A Practical Guide', which draws upon the work of Professor Ian Cumming, will show how management theory can be applied at many different levels to the perioperative setting.

The key message from this book is to encourage those staff already working as leaders and managers in perioperative practice to engage further with principles and theories that relate directly to the care of patients. For those staff currently studying leadership and management, this book will prove a valuable resource to aid progress and will provide opportunities to reflect on current knowledge and understanding of a number of contemporary issues embedded in perioperative care.

It is not our claim that the chapters in this book cover every aspect of the professional life of a perioperative leader and manager. Rather we have as far as possible addressed the most pressing contemporary topics that are prevalent in today's perioperative environment. The book has been specifically written for perioperative practitioners who are seeking to build and consolidate their management and leadership skills, both practical and theoretical.

**Brian Smith, Paul Rawling,
Paul Wicker, Chris Jones**

Managing change in perioperative education

Brian Smith

Key Learning Points

- Explore the key milestones in perioperative education
- Define some of the conflicts and tensions that occurred
- Discuss new ways of teaching and learning in perioperative education

The purpose of this chapter is to highlight the confusion, conflicts and challenges faced by many academic staff and staff involved with perioperative education. To appreciate the changes that have occurred, this chapter will navigate through the key milestones in perioperative education, offering an insight into how they have provided a road map of today's perioperative education.

Operating department assistant training

From 1976 and until the 1990s, education for the operating department assistant and the operating department practitioner (ODP) was available through regional training centres. The City and Guilds of London Institute approved the regional training centres following recommendations made by the Lewin Report (Department of Health 1970). This offered many recruits, who came from diverse backgrounds and who did not always have perioperative experience, an opportunity to enter into perioperative practice.

The course itself comprised of two calendar years where the 'trainee ODA' was exposed to specialities within the theatre suite. Trainees were also invited to visit other departments that had a direct influence on their perioperative work. For some, visiting accident & emergency, sterile services, coronary care and intensive care units expanded their knowledge and understanding of medicine and healthcare.

Managing this programme was not straightforward. Day-to-day coordination of ODA's training and welfare resided with the local assessment coordinator (LAC) or local assessment manager (LAM). The person performing this role was either from a theatre nursing or an ODA background. The two different names – LAC and LAM – resulted in tensions and conflict. That is, the LAMs viewed their role as a managerial one as opposed to being a coordinator of the City and Guilds' programme. The perceived difference between the two names occurred because of different expectations of the role within clinical practice. Anecdotal evidence at the time suggested the LAMs were recruited because of their seniority in the operating theatres and were expected to line manage the trainee too. However, the regional centre guidance for the LAC's role included the perioperative practitioner (not necessarily in a senior position) designing, implementing and evaluating the training programme. The manager in charge of the operating theatres line managed the trainee.

Core Topics in Operating Department Practice: Leadership and Management, ed. Brian Smith, Paul Rawling, Paul Wicker and Chris Jones. Published by Cambridge University Press. © Cambridge University Press 2010.

Although LAC job descriptions were available, the LAM title continued to be used in several hospitals. We can assume the existence of the two titles may have occurred because of personnel seeking to progress their career or as a result of organic change as the programme developed. Nevertheless, the existence of the LAC & LAM titles continued to create tension for the learner and the perioperative staff. There were examples of how the confusing titles did affect the learning experience, either positively and negatively. For example, the LAM often provided an authoritative voice, ensuring the student gained access to placements. However, the LAC offered pastoral support, guidance and direction for the student. As the LAC was not responsible for the day-to-day management of the trainee's behaviour, attitudes and work ethics, the relationship between the trainee and LAC may have been more sympathetic. Often, trainees felt they could approach their LAC with emotional difficulties. Some felt they were unable to approach the LAM and preferred to consult a LAC, who acted independently from any managerial demands. Moreover, the LAM's managerial position may have aggravated the situation. That is, within the nature of management, there is a need for the manager to have some 'control' over staff performance and how it aligns with the service delivery (Tannenbaum 1968: 3). Control within this context is not restrictive or oppression of an individual's autonomy or capabilities, but is one where the trainee ODA is motivated and inspired to learn by performing healthcare activities that are within their scope of practice and which meet the organization's purpose. The LAC role, at the time, did offer stimulus for the trainee to learn new competencies in many areas of anaesthesia, surgery and recovery. Nevertheless, LACs were also faced with trainee ODAs 'failing to progress' or underperforming. The 'control' element would have tried to influence poor performance and undesirable behaviour to encourage progress. The LAM role would have a certain amount of responsibility to manage this, whereas the LAC would have referred the problem to their line manager or the regional centre. Given that the

two titles existed, trainee ODAs often became confused, leaving them to undertake a complex and demanding programme along with trying to make sense of who was supporting them; was it the LAC or the LAM?

Irrespective of the LAC or LAM dilemma, the regional management of the hospital ODA qualification from the City and Guilds of London Institute involved the regional health authorities. They became responsible for the regional training centre as it was funded from public money collected by the UK Government. The managerial structure of the programme included a local steering group, which was sometimes referred to as the local management committee. The membership of this group included ODAs, nurses, anaesthetists and surgeons, with representatives from hospitals in the area. These senior colleagues were given the responsibility to ensure that the National Health Service Training Authority standards were integrated alongside the course syllabus. Again there was some disjointedness in the names applied to this group; however, the benefit of having a steering group meant that rigorous scrutiny of the programmes ensured that they were fit for purpose and did, in fact, make a difference to the patient and the trainee's experience. Although City and Guilds of London Institute was primarily responsible for quality assurance, the local steering groups also saw their role as quality assurors of the course. Managing quality assurance is something that needs significant thought and does need a dedicated body of experts to question what they implement. This also applies to any perioperative practitioners under their related codes of conduct (Health Professions Council and Nursing and Midwifery Council). Indeed LACs were champions of quality, which was seen in the highly effective training packages that they provided for the trainee ODA. The quality was measured through the high success rate of the programme and the high volume of applicants wishing to train in their hospital. The reputation of good ODA training spread across the country, thus promoting the new profession.

Given that ODA training was successful, many have asked why there was a need for change. There was some controversy with how the trainee ODA was assessed during the programme. The assessment included a multiple-choice questionnaire examination and two practical assessments: anaesthesia assistance and surgical scrubbing. A report of 'good' trainees passing the practical and failing the examination was seen as unfair. That is, the trainee who excelled in practice and did not cope with examination pressures was seen as disadvantaged because there was too much emphasis on the theoretical element. Furthermore, in 1989, the Department of Health published the Bevan Report, which investigated the utilization and management of operating theatres (NHS Management Executive VFM Unit 1989). Changing UK demographics in health were placing more demands on healthcare, and the study helped to identify where and how healthcare could be improved. Professor P. G. Bevan led the study and later recommended that the nurse education body (English National Board (ENB)) and the National Health Service Training Directorate (NHSTD; formerly the National Health Service Training Authority) should work collaboratively to develop a common training programme for theatre staff. He recognized that there was much commonality in what nursing and ODA staff studied during their education. The report also recommended that 'levels of competence' should be ascertained for each role in the operating department so the boundaries of professional practice, the division of labour, were clear. Sharing knowledge was seen as good practice and it was hoped that this would lead to greater harmony among the professions.

Perioperative nursing programmes

For several years, the ENB offered specialist courses for registered nurses (RN) to develop their knowledge and skills: ENB 176 Operating Department Practice Award, ENB 182 Anaesthetic Nursing and ENB 183 Anaesthetic and Theatre Award. The ENB qualifications for the operating department became UK recognized. The 'theatre course' was much sought after, with many nurses leaving their home towns to undertake the course. The theatre course focused on skill acquisition and was supported heavily by testing the nurses' understanding through course work. As Brett (1996) has previously explained, these courses migrated into higher education, offering opportunities for the RN to achieve a diploma or degree pathway in theatre nursing. Reshaping of the ENB courses led to topics such as ethics and research skills becoming important in the curriculum. This resulted in a reduction of time previously earmarked for specialities such as anaesthesia. This caused controversy among the nursing staff and concern from the ODA profession. There were claims that the new short courses were inadequate to teach the full range of skills, thus not producing the 'knowledgeable doer'. Disagreement over this issue followed, with conflict growing between the ODA and nursing groups.

Conflict is unavoidable in any organization where multiprofessional groups operate, as one group will have a different paradigm to another. While conflict itself cannot be avoided, any adverse effects that might occur can be managed, and as a result, this was a time of great activity in theatre management, and debate in the perioperative literature. Many theatre managers tried to clarify the objectives of the service. Educators involved in both programmes delivered conference presentations and journal articles, or found other ways to clarify the misunderstandings. With any organizational conflict, Mullins (1999) tells us that there are several strategies that can be used. One key strategy that can work for the operating department is to develop interpersonal and group process skills. This approach encourages everyone to communicate their viewpoint and become involved in developing constructive solutions to the conflict. This approach may work if the issue is restricted to organizational levels. Given that the conflict between the ODA and nurse was national and in many organizations, then an independent body needed to intervene.

Introduction of the operating department practitioner role

The Bevan Report (NHS Management Executive VFM Unit 1989) was timely in identifying the issues among the groups working in the operating department, giving hope that the changes would be worthwhile for all.

The Bevan Report was a catalyst for the new generation of theatre worker, the ODP. The ODP role was not intended to replace the traditional roles of the nurse and ODA. Instead, the ODP was envisaged to have the appropriate skills and knowledge to move between different theatre situations and perform alongside colleagues in anaesthesia, recovery and surgery.

At the time this role was developed, tension grew between many nursing and ODA staff. It was common knowledge that a divide existed between the two groups, with most of the ODA staff remaining in the specialist area of anaesthesia. Assisting the surgeon became the home place for RNs, with few moving into the anaesthetic field. At times, this division caused disputes and unsatisfactory working conditions for both groups, resulting in 'bad feelings'. Some managers adopted an autocratic style of managing, providing limited opportunity for staff consultation and resulting in the issue intensifying. While it is recognized that the different management styles of autocratic, democratic, consultative and laissez-faire are commonly covered in education and training sessions, the adoption of any one style is at the discretion of the user. An autocratic style of theatre management is not something that is necessarily taught or advocated during training sessions but it may develop as an automatic response to the 'flight, fright and fight' pressure that managers face. This is discussed further in Ch. 8.

Introducing the ODP role further exacerbated the divisions and tensions between the ODA and the nurse. Many ODAs and nurses were unsure of which group the ODP belonged to and, therefore, engaged in further arguments of who should manage the ODP. Underlying this was a feeling that the ODP would take jobs from nurses wishing to enter theatres following their basic training. The ODAs were concerned that the ODP would be a cheap replacement for them, even though ODAs had always been trained in anaesthesia, surgery and patient care. Both groups had their concerns and entered a battle for control for ODP alliances. Belbin's (1993) discussion about teams at work shows that there are different types of individual within teams, which can also be inherent within groups. In this situation, where the new member, the ODP, does not yet belong within either group or team, there will be courtship towards the individual to become a member of one of the other groups. This occurs unless a new group forms with sufficient membership to maintain its existence.

Introducing national vocational training

As the new role was introduced, the Department of Health also recommended that a vocational training package should be made available for operating department staff. This was part of a wider remit to offer vocational qualifications across the UK for equipping the workforce with correct skills and knowledge. A new governing organization was formed, the National Council for Vocational Qualifications (NCVQ), to approve these new qualifications.

For the operating department, the NCVQ drew on the expertise of the Care Sector Consortium (now referred to as Skills for Health) to write the occupational standards. Experts from the consortium produced the new standards, which later influenced the City and Guilds of London Institute and other providers offering the 'National Vocation Qualification (NVQ) in Health Care: Operating Department Practice Level 3' award. This award was intended to supersede the City and Guilds of London Institute 752 award for the ODA and the ENB certificate for 'theatre practice'. This caused disruption between the two professions, as some believed the vocational programme would devalue their hard-earned qualification. Media coverage and the comparison by both professions of the new qualification to other NVQ awards, such as hairdressing, were perceived as insulting to their professions. Some predicted that future employment of theatre staff would only be for those with the Operating Department Practice Level 3 NVQ Award. Despite several attempts to clarify and lessen the anxiety of perioperative staff, they remained unconvinced and disheartened with the future of perioperative practice. Disharmony between the managers and the staff caused local and perhaps a national trend of ODAs and nurses seeking other employment. For many, joining an agency was much more attractive as they were not governed by any one manager and the salary was more lucrative.

As the number of ODAs and nurses leaving to join an agency grew, the perioperative service faced several challenges. Day-to-day management of operating lists required the team leader (or person in charge) to pay closer attention to skill mix, the resources available (staff and equipment) and to any disruption in work flow. That is, if a delay occurred when transferring a patient from the ward to the operating theatre, the time and reason was noted and later reported in a departmental meeting. Audits too were conducted to identify time wasted because of delays, staff sickness, lack of equipment and other reasons. Managing this change required a new set of skills by the team leader, and some undertook an academic course of study. The importance of leadership and management were mentioned in the *NHS Plan* (Department of Health 2000), which advocated that leadership and managerial skills were something that all grades of staff should acquire. Furthermore, increased authority to make appropriate decisions within their job role empowered the manager to improve working conditions, job satisfaction and patient care.

Most higher education institutions offer generic and discipline-specific leadership and management courses. Perioperative staff have inherently chosen the health-related leadership programmes. Those attending these programmes were exposed to many theoretical models of leadership and management. Problem-based learning, with examples of good and bad leadership, aided the learner in appreciating how to manage the complexities of running an operating list.

For the LAC or other educators involved in the new ODP training, the differentials that emerged during recruitment of the 'trainee ODP' caused confusion. The NVQ concept of training was that it was open to all students irrespective of sex, sexual orientation, race, religion or creed, and that the training should not be bound by time. The belief that the trainee does not 'fail' but simply does 'not achieve' the skill, knowledge or attitude required of the function encourages individuals to continue to try to succeed. This was not adhered to as most employers restricted the timescale by using training contracts. The employer would require successful candidates to agree and sign a two-year training contract. If the individual had not completed the course after the two-year period, he or she could be considered for an extension. Some individuals were unsuccessful in obtaining an extension and did not complete their Operating Department Practice Award. Naturally, when this occurred for the unfortunate few, the LAC would have been involved either in the decision making or after the event with pastoral support. The decision not to continue with a trainee ODP would have been taken through a thorough process, looking at achievements, retention of knowledge, general demeanour and suitability for perioperative practice. The LAC would have provided information and given their account of the individual's abilities. Following this decision, the LAC would have provided emotional support for those who perceive they had 'failed'. In this situation, the LAC would have used counselling skills, such as active listening and paraphrasing to assist the individual to make sense of the outcome. Not all LACs had undertaken learning about counselling skills and, therefore, relied on their own thoughts on how to offer emotional support. This is a particular area where access to further education for staff in this role could have strengthened the quality of support provided.

Likewise, the work-based trainers and assessors may have felt that they had failed in their duties in helping the trainee to gather enough evidence proving their competence. Anecdotal evidence at the time from work-based assessor meetings indicate how involved the work-based assessor became with the trainee's progress. If a fail occurred, many reflected on their activities and wondered how they could have improved the opportunities for the trainee. Although there were elements of reflection in their practice, the reflective cycle of Gibbs, Kolb, Driscoll and others were not necessarily in use. This came much later as the ODP award progressed into higher education.

In any award, be it NVQ or higher education, there are internal and external quality assurances that ensure that the learner's achievements have met national standards. Within the NVQ structure, the guardians of these were the internal and external verifiers. Rigorous scrutiny of the trainee's work took place and it was then 'signed off' by the external verifier. This report triggered the final process within the City and Guilds London Institute by awarding the certificate of achievement. This is similar to what takes place today in universities.

Moving into higher education

During the 1990s, the ODP programme took a leap of faith into higher education as the polytechnics were being reshaped and becoming universities. From the mid 1990s, universities offering the ODP NVQ Level 3 Award also offered a Certificate of Higher Education in the ODP programme. The dual award gave the recently renamed student ODP (formerly trainee ODP) recognition of the detailed knowledge and practice the ODP was expected to attain. Likewise, the change of status from trainee to student was a mark of acceptance that their studies were not just vocational but also academic.

The dual award ran for almost five years until a campaign led by the Association of Operating Department Practice came to fruition in 2001,

where the new ODP award was the Diploma of Higher Education in Operating Department Practice. This award, and accepting ODPs as a profession by the Health Professions Council in 2004, meant that their new award would face further scrutiny.

Today, universities offer ODPs access to higher education awards, such as diplomas, first degrees and masters. As the ODP award became set within higher education, many universities managed applications themselves. However, as the Department of Health increased the funding made available to universities, there was a rise in numbers of student ODPs. The larger cohorts required new systems and processes to keep up with demand. This meant organization change in how applications were processed. The application process for the Pre-registration Diploma in Operating Department Practice is similar to the nursing pre-registration programme administered by the central body, the Universities and Colleges Admissions Service (UCAS). Their service provides students with information to make the correct informed choice about their health career. Moving ODP applications to this service removed any subjective elements to the recruitment process that may have existed previously.

Recruitment of qualified ODP and nurses to post-registration courses (i.e. the degree and master programmes in perioperative practice) is managed internally by the university. This is often devolved to faculty or college level, where the numbers of students are often much lower.

Previously, the central team for ODP training carried out administrative duties and teaching, the change in application process has meant that the teaching staff is free to enrich the student learning experience. This change may be straightforward but changes in an organization's systems or process evoke different responses within and from individuals.

Changes in any system should be initiated by first considering what you wish to change and why. In the example above, the desire to change the application process to UCAS was primarily to show parity between professional groups: the nurses and ODPs. A second reason included the rise in student ODP numbers and the demand this would have placed on teaching staff time.

When viewing the advantages of change, we must consider who it will affect and how they might react to it. Any change should ideally have a 'win–win' situation, where all affected by the change will benefit.

Mode neutral approaches to operating department practitioner education

Further changes are afoot as many universities continue to break new ground into learning, teaching and e-learning research. Given that the National Health Service (NHS) has a strong e-learning strategy and values the flexibility of developing staff without removing them from the clinical setting, universities continue to explore and invest into blended and online learning.

Orthodox classroom teaching often involves an academic providing a linear and didactic approach to transferring knowledge to the student (ODPs and nurses). This style of teaching and learning is referred to as instructivism. Absorbing the ideas or directives from those delivering the session has been through repetition either in clinical skills laboratories or within the clinical setting. It can be argued that in healthcare it is necessary to appreciate what is best practice in order to lessen the risk of a patient being harmed. Indeed, this is paramount to the learner's practice; however, the internalization of the repeated events does not necessarily show deep levels of cognition. It has been claimed that the student merely memorizes sequences or responses to the situation in instructivist learning cultures. They may respond to a question or clinical situation; however, most recall the detail without making sense of what they have learnt.

The alternative, which is gaining popularity, is constructivist learning and teaching. Instead of students being passive recipients, they are expected to actively construct their knowledge and ideas from interaction with others and drawing on resources. Inherent within this style of facilitating learning, there are elements where the student can reflect and deconstruct their understanding of a particular matter. This can occur in any 'learning space', such as the classroom, online or in the clinical setting. The key difference here is how the academic and clinical staff act as a resource rather than a source of knowledge. Increasingly within the digital society there is a harnessing of collective intelligence, where one learns from another, and this offers greater opportunity for deeper learning to take place. The work of Smith, who incidentally is a perioperative practitioner, has stimulated a new wave in learning and teaching not only for perioperative staff but also for other disciplines through publishing principles of teaching and learning known as 'mode neutral pedagogy' (Smith *et al.* 2008).

Mode neutral was first hypothesized in 2006, where the creator tested the theory with post-registration students; theatre nurses and ODPs studying anaesthesia and/or recovery. The teaching and learning experience in mode neutral is designed to embrace each learner's characteristics, as described by Landsberger (2004:8): 'learners increasingly will be from different backgrounds. They will desire and require flexibility in the ways that they study, the resources they use, the sorts of activities that they do and the ways in which they interact and communicate.'

Therefore, 'Mode Neutral is a method that allows students to progress across modes of delivery at any point throughout their study when their preferences, requirements, personal and professional commitments demand, without compromising their learning experience' (Smith *et al.* 2008).

One research study found that there was greater connection within the clinical setting using this method, suggesting that the much-acclaimed theory-to-practice gap in nursing (Landers 2000) was, in fact, closing (Smith & Rawling 2008:191). Similarly, Smith & Rawling (2008) reported how a mixed group of learners, ODPs and nurses, interacting online or in the classroom, were breaking down barriers and working collaboratively.

The findings of Smith and colleagues have brought insight into how perioperative education can be reconceptualized to offer *freedom to explore and learn* without causing any risk to the patient. Although mode neutral pedagogy is not fully discussed here, in short the key principles are:

1. Encouraging the learner to own and control how they learn
2. Modes of learning are more prevalent than modes of delivery
3. Harnessing collective intelligence enriches personal learning
4. A flexible single learning space encourages a single community of practice.

Given that this new pedagogy differs from traditional methods of delivering perioperative education, some challenges may be faced by students, staff and the organizations.

A student of perioperative practice with a previous educational experience involving conditioning to be recipients of information may find that internal adjustments have to be made to the new experience. As one of the mode neutral principles suggests, the student (learner) will own and control their learning: that is, they will have autonomy to seek out information rather than wait to be given it. By shifting the 'Locus of Control' (Rotter 1996), they can learn in multiple ways outwith the classroom environment. That is, the use of their own digital technology (mobile phone, MP3 players, computers) and that made available by the universities will encourage continual learning at times convenient to the student.

Similarly, academic and perioperative staff using digital forms or conventional forms of teaching will have to reconcile to the fact that they are no longer the 'controllers' of knowledge information. Instead, they act as one of many sources of specialist knowledge that the student can draw on. Mode neutral style of teaching will also place demands on staff to create closer alignment of theory with practice. This involves fostering effective conditions within the learning space (physical and virtual) for the student to become involved in communication for learning.

Within the clinical setting, the change that would be necessary to promote an effective learning experience is to gain access to the 'academic' curriculum. That is, academics, clinical and mentoring staff should have an identical view to the perioperative student. Mode neutral offers this view by presenting the curriculum through a single learning space; a virtual learning environment or other social and content management systems. Campus sessions can be recorded and archived within the space, offering an opportunity for learning to be extended beyond the traditional classroom session. For the perioperative staff supporting the learner, this means that they can assist with integrating the student's knowledge into clinical practice by using the virtual learning environment as a teaching resource. Discussions in the clinical setting may also occur from the online activities, leading into a sense of shared learning among the operating team, including medical colleagues.

For this new approach in perioperative education to continue successfully, perioperative practitioners will need to develop closer affinities with the universities and this will provide encouragement and direction for becoming effective mentors. That is, such staff will be able to see how their contribution has a significant part to play in deepening the knowledge, skills and attitudes of the student in perioperative practice.

Furthermore, the university embracing mode neutral to enrich the student experience will provide the appropriate resources (human and digital) so that students can exercise their learning wherever and whenever they want. This will place demand on the academic rigour for supporting and encouraging student progression.

Conclusions

Perioperative education has faced and conquered many challenges since the late 1970s. The continuous reshaping of health education has brought many benefits to the student, the provider and the health service; however this does not mean that the current programmes (pre- and post-registration) are without any flaws. The health demographics in the UK population do change and this creates challenges not only for the health service but also for providers of health education. As the health service continues to find new ways of working to meet new demands, researchers in higher education methods investigate the impact of such education within healthcare. Their search to discover new ways of teaching and learning, as well as subject-specific links between poor and good health, provide timely education. This means that they can provide education that enriches the learner's experience but they also realize that there will never be a 'perfect' programme because of the continual changes in health matters. Moreover, they realize that providing a flexible experience that stimulates the practitioner to embrace their learning and to use that knowledge as a scaffold will lead these practitioners to become 'fit for purpose'.

This chapter has considered key milestones in the timeline of perioperative education that have caused confusion, conflict and challenges requiring management. Those who have dealt with these milestones during the ODA and ENB training have provided a legacy for future generations of perioperative staff in clinical, academic or researcher roles to draw upon when searching for new ways of aligning theory with practice and of enriching the perioperative student experience. For some, accepting change can cause internal conflict; however, reconciling and embracing the change may offer a more collaborative and personally satisfying experience. Ultimately, it will show that perioperative practitioners who continue to adopt an evidence-based approach to their practice will offer their patients a high quality of care.

REFERENCES

Belbin, M. (1993). *Team Roles at Work*. Oxford: Butterworth/Heinemann.

Brett, M. (1996). Educating theatre nurses: a framework for the future. *Nursing Standard*, **11**, 50–51.

Department of Health (1970). *Organisation and Staffing of Operating Departments [Lewin Report]*. London: The Stationery Office.

Department of Health (2000). *The NHS Plan: A Plan for Investment, a Plan for Reform*. London: The Stationery Office; http://www.dh.gov.uk/en/Publicationsandstatistics/Publications/PublicationsPolicyandGuidance/DH_4002960 (accessed 10 October 2008).

Landers, M.G. (2000). The theory–practice gap in nursing: the role of the nurse teacher. *Journal of Advanced Nursing*, **32**, 1550–1557.

Landsberger, J. (2004). E-learning by design: an interview with Dr Betty Collis. *TechTrends*, **48**, 7–12.

Mullins, L. (1999). *Management and Organisational Behaviour*, 5th edn. Edinburgh: Pearson Education.

NHS Management Executive VFM Unit (1989). *Staffing and Utilisation of Operating Theatres: A Study Conducted Under the Guidance of a Steering Group [Bevan Report]*. Leeds: NHS Management Executive VFM Unit.

Rotter, J. (1966). Generalized expectancies for internal versus external control of reinforcements. *Psychological Monographs*, **80**, 609.

Smith, B. & Rawling, P. (2008). Anaesthetic assistant competencies: our experience. *Journal of Perioperative Practice*, **18**, 190–192.

Smith, B., Reed, P. & Jones, C. (2008). Mode neutral pedagogy. *European Journal of Open and Distance Learning (EURODL)*; http://www.eurodl.org/materials/contrib/2008/Smith_Reed_Jones.htm (accessed 10 October 2008).

Tannenbaum, A.S. (1968). *Control in Organizations*. New York: McGraw-Hill.

2

The role of the operating department manager within the context of the organization

Paul Wicker

Key Learning Points
- Explore the role of the manager
- Define the roles and functions of management
- Discuss organizational structure and function.

The purpose of this chapter is to introduce some of the concepts associated with management in the context of the operating department, the hospital and the health service. Management is management, wherever it is carried out. But operating department management is special because of the context of patient care, the management needs of diverse groups of staff and the challenging environment, distinctive by its high technology, fast pace and constantly changing requirements. This chapter introduces some of these challenges for the operating department manager by looking at the context in which managers work, what managers do and why they do it.

What comes to mind when thinking about management? Some of the key concepts are shown in Table 2.1.

According to Koontz & Weihrich (1990), management is the process of designing and maintaining an environment in which individuals work together in groups efficiently to accomplish their goals or aims. These principles apply at all levels of hierarchy in an organization. The role of the manager is, therefore, concerned with increasing productivity, effectiveness and efficiency. It is the art, or science, of 'getting things done'. In the operating department, this can be identified as ensuring the maximum numbers of patients are treated safely and quickly and that the best treatment is delivered in the best way, with the least cost. To do this, the manager has to coordinate and integrate the department's activities through planning, organizing, directing and controlling resources to achieve patient expectations and to accomplish their specific departmental goals and objectives (Sullivan & Decker 1988).

Aside from these functions, Mintzberg (1973) suggests that managers also have to perform several roles. For example, in the course of a day, a manager might have to be a figurehead (such as inspiring the team to do a better job), a leader (guiding the team through a difficult situation) or a liaison (acting as a link between surgeons, anaesthetists, practitioners and ward staff). At the same time, the manager will also have to manage the flow of information within the organization, for example receiving information (about an operating list), disseminating information (about a patient's procedure) or acting as a spokesperson (at a meeting). And of course the manager has to be a decision maker, adopting the role of entrepreneur (e.g. identifying opportunities, encouraging and initiating change), allocating resources (rostering staff) and negotiating (discounts on purchases of equipment). Add to this the never ending task of dealing with the sometimes conflicting needs of other managers, patients, surgeons, anaesthetists, operating

Core Topics in Operating Department Practice: Leadership and Management, ed. Brian Smith, Paul Rawling, Paul Wicker and Chris Jones. Published by Cambridge University Press. © Cambridge University Press 2010.

Table 2.1 Key concepts in management

Area	Concepts
The organisation	Structure
	Function
	Authority
	Accountability
	Hierarchy
The functions of the manager	Planning
	Organizing
	Directing
	Controlling
	Staffing
	Budgeting
The roles of the manager	Productivity
	Leadership
	Power
	Delegation
	Efficiency
	Effectiveness

department practitioners and nurses, and it is little wonder that the operating department manager's job is sometimes cited as challenging, demanding, onerous, thankless, exciting and rewarding – amongst others!

Managers are charged with the responsibility for taking actions that will maximize the contribution of each member of the organization. The goal of management is, therefore, to increase the productivity of the organization (Mintzberg *et al.* 1998). In an operating department, this means achieving higher utilization of operating rooms and treating more patients, with the least number of staff possible. This situation is balanced by the need for safety and quality; for example, checking accountable items during a surgical procedure may be enforced even though it slows down the operating list. The overall result sought is still increased efficiency and effectiveness of the department.

So, is management an art or a science? In some ways it is both. The way a manager develops is the sum of the individual's experience and education or training. Experiential learning is acquired by people

in different ways – what is a learning experience to one will completely pass over the head of another. In addition, the range of experiences that are experienced by the time a practitioner is ready to become a manager is so vast as to be indescribable. Finally, the element of creativity, the ability to see things differently from everybody else, is also unique to each individual.

So is there really a need for a creative manager? As the world of art has shown us, creativity exists in every aspect of life (Thinkexist 2008), from a tin of beans to a rusty iron angel standing in a field – and maybe creativity even exists in the decision-making processes of an operating department manager. So perhaps the way managers practise, the nuances of their daily work and the jigsaw of daily decision making, is, in fact, an art that is unique to the individual. However, it is an art with a scientific core, supported by an increasingly complex knowledge base. This unique combination of art and science is what makes each manager's approach to management unique – and what makes some managers merely acceptable, while others excel.

Organizational structure and function

An organization is a framework within which people in various groups carry out activities (Meeker & Rothrock 1991). The purpose of an organization is to enable the workers to carry out these activities more efficiently than they could do if working alone. Organizations work within each other; hence the operating department works within the hospital, which works within the NHS. A huge amount of organization theory has developed to help to explain the way organizations work (Mintzberg *et al.* 1998). The modern day NHS is very different to the old NHS; it is more flexible, more responsive to change and much more efficient and effective. This has been achieved through a huge investment in resources and massive and continual changes since its inception (NHS Education Scotland 2008).

One way in which organizations can keep up with change and 'stay ahead of the game' is through strategy formation (Mintzberg *et al.* 1998). The way that an organization works is often dependent on the approach to developing its strategy (Hatch, 1997). While a hospital's strategy is likely to be published widely in a 'glossy' document, a department's strategy is more likely to be implied in the way policies, procedures, committees and projects are operated, and the way managers manage people.

The classical approach to management is the oldest and most influential (Whittington 1993). It heavily depends on a rational approach to decision making and analysis and quantification of the various factors influencing the organization. The rational approach has often been used in the past because of the clear and logical approach taken. However, while the classical model encourages the generation of hard data to underpin developments, it is less able to account for unpredictable and sudden changes in practice or knowledge, which will require several innovative approaches to develop to address the change (Hatch 1997). For example, consider the difficulties with introducing swab racks, universal precautions and quality assurance in the early 1970s and the 1980s. The classical approach to management valued stability, whereas the revolutionary ideas being introduced at the time required explosive and ongoing change. The classical model is also unable to take account of the cultural values in the organization. Both these factors are very important in today's NHS, where change occurs almost daily and the workforce comprises several groups of highly trained, influential workers. Hence the classical model of management, while still enduring, is rapidly being replaced by more flexible and dynamic approaches.

The Cultural School sees the approach to management developing as a result of social interaction based on the beliefs and understandings of the organization's members (Mintzberg *et al.* 1998). The manager subscribes to the organization's culture, and vice versa. One advantage of this approach is that resistance to change is likely to be reduced because the need for change (that is, the role of managers to manage) is supported by its members (Burnes 2004). A negative aspect is that a strong culture might encourage a status quo because people on the whole would rather avoid change, especially change with a negative impact on their own situations (Scott & Jaffe 1989, Burnes 2004). The culture of the operating department impacts on the way that it works, particularly in regard to recruitment and retention of staff, the way staff are managed and the use of resources (Bate 2002). For example, a dictatorial manager is more likely to support an arrogant and overbearing surgeon, and a staff composed of forward thinking and dynamic members is more likely to require 'light touch' management. It is likely, therefore, that the management of departments or hospitals will be aligned in some way or other to the Cultural School model.

Followers of the Learning School believe that every informed member of an organization takes part in developing their organization as they learn about the situation they are in (Mintzberg *et al.* 1998). A learning organization is one where there is constant change and developments as its members learn how to manage changing situations. The learning organization values individual learning, which contributes to the overall organizational aims and objectives. This approach takes account of the fact that life is not rational or linear, and that those who are closest to the customer (or the patient) may be best placed to effect worthwhile change. While this approach to management might seem likely in the operating department, given the high numbers of learned professionals working there, it appears to have little use in an environment where only a small amount of time is set aside for dialogue and debate, and precedence is given to quick decisions and action taking. Nevertheless, a learning organization is seen as being valuable and managers should do their best to ensure that their organization is influenced by this model.

Williams and Tse (1995) believe that the entrepreneurial approach is one where there is a strong leader, who usually makes the key decisions.

The leader is charismatic and often highly effective at leading an organization down a particular path. Many operating department managers adopt an approach like this, because of the need to respond quickly to changes in the internal and external environments of their department. To a certain extent, this type of manager reflects Williams and Tse's (1995) 'opportunistic entrepreneur' who is characterized by a leader with a middle-class background, who is well educated formally and who has broad work experiences. Such a leader favours decentralized management and is highly orientated towards the future, following developments in the service and focusing on output and efficiency as key measures of success.

There are many ways to think of the management and organization of an operating department, and these are just a few of them. What is clear, though, is that the way the operating department works, its culture, management ethos and its strategy affect the way its workers work with each other, and the way patient care is delivered. The operating department manager is a key influence on the underlying strategies employed by the department to achieve its goals. This is discussed further in Chs. 6 and 12.

Organizational structure

Every organization has a chain of command, or a hierarchy. This is especially clear in an operating department, which has a long history of a 'pecking order'. Officially, the operating department manager is in charge of staff, resources, the day-to-day operation of the service and its ongoing development. However, the reality is more complex because other groups also have a say in the way the department runs. The surgeon, for example, may insist on operating on a particular patient first, or an anaesthetist may make a demand for a particular level of practitioner to assist him or her in the anaesthetic room. Similarly, an experienced practitioner may refuse to work in a particular way if he or she feels that it compromises their patient's care.

Managing the informal culture, by an approach to leadership, may, therefore, be one of the most important roles of the manager in the operating department (Ch. 8).

The chain of command is a path of authority and accountability from one person to another: every person in an organization has a manager within the organization, apart from the chief executive or chairman, who often will have their managers outside the organization. The different layers of the chain of authority are represented by post holders. Normally, the management roles of those at the bottom of the chain are less complex than those at the top of the chain. So, for example, while a practitioner in an operating room may be responsible for allocating the workload for the day, a clinical manager may be responsible for allocating the staff in all the operating rooms. Furthermore, an operating department manager will be responsible for ensuring that all resources are available, and also that the service develops in response to changing needs of the users. Consequently, the span of control of managers, and their influence over the strategic direction of the organization, increases as they climb the hierarchy (Hatch 1997). The ultimate control normally lodges with the chief executive, who has a corporate responsibility for the entire organization. This concept is discussed further in Ch. 6.

Levels of management

There are three recognized categories of managers: top level, middle level and first level.

Top-level managers are responsible for strategically managing and guiding the organization as a whole. The posts have titles such as chief executive, chief operational officer, chief nurse and director of nursing. They recognize and respond to internal and external influences and are able to make decisions that have few guidelines because they often move into new territory where decisions have not been made before. Leaders at this level are more

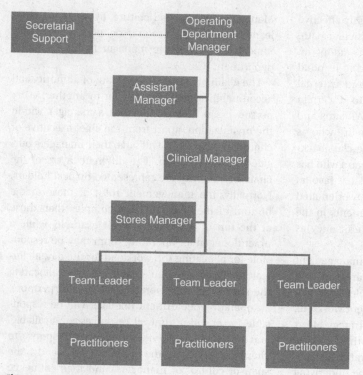

Figure 2.1 A simple organization chart for an operating department.

concerned with 'strategy' than 'operational' measures and so do not get caught up in the minutiae of daily living. They determine the philosophy of the organization, the strategic direction and they create goals and priorities for resource allocation. Post holders in these positions usually have excellent leadership and interpersonal skills as they have to lead and inspire their organization to move in new directions or to take certain paths.

Middle-level managers coordinate the roles of the lower levels on the hierarchy. They act as a conduit for information between the lower levels and the higher levels. Their roles include day-to-day operations, long-term planning, establishing unit policies and managing staff. They, therefore, have a foot in each camp: on one side are the workers doing the day-to-day work of an organization and on the other side are the upper level managers who oversee the strategic direction of the organization. Examples of middle managers

are nurse supervisors, head nurses, unit managers, business managers and administration managers. Many middle managers see their positions as difficult because of tension between the lower and the upper parts of the organization. Such is the life of the middle manager!

The first-level managers are usually concerned with specific unit work flow and they deal with immediate problems with daily operations. Examples of first-level managers are charge nurses, team leaders and coordinators.

Most organizations, and some operating departments, have organization charts to represent their formal structure, the post holders and the relationships between them (Fig. 2.1).

An organization chart is useful for visualizing the structure of an organization quickly; however, it does have its limitations. For example, it does not show informal relationships (such as managers from different departments who have similar interests); neither can it illustrate the degree of responsibility or authority for each level. It is also · at risk of becoming obsolete quickly, since some departments seem to change annually in response to changing workload or environment.

An organization chart can also show the type of organizational structure that is used by the department. The following discussion looks at two of the main types of structure: tall or centralized, and flat or decentralized.

A tall or centralized organization allocates decision-making authority and power to people in a few central positions. The typical operating department structure follows this model. For example, the operating department manager is at the top of the hierarchy, followed by a deputy, a selection of team leaders and then the practitioners. The assistants often do not line-manage staff and are not part of the centralized structure. Therefore, an assistant to an operating department manager will not necessarily be the natural successor to the post if the manager leaves. The structure will be supported by others, such as secretaries, who are not part of the formal structure themselves. The persons in authority are responsible only for those directly below them, usually small in number, and the structure is likely to have many levels.

Centralized structures such as this benefit from providing close supervision to subordinates; therefore, less-skilled individuals can be supported well. Additionally, individuals in key positions can also show and develop their expertise because there are fewer of them (on that level) compared with other structures and so they stand out more: their decision making, for example, is more visible. Top managers are spared from unnecessary communication because it can be dealt with by subordinates, and those at the top have a great deal of power to delegate tasks and activities down the levels. There are several disadvantages. For example, skilled individuals may be stifled and restricted by the close control of their manager, therefore reducing their contribution to the department (Hatch 1997). Communication normally only travels up and down the structure from one level to the next. This

can take a long time, if it is impeded at any stage, and this may delay the implementation of decisions. For example, a decision to change practice may be quickly made by a group of practitioners but may then be delayed for weeks if a line manager is on holiday.

Traditional hospital structures adopt this type of structure, although its inflexibility and inability to handle complex and rapidly changing situations have forced hospital managers to move towards other structures.

A flat or decentralized structure has fewer levels and a broader span of control since decision making is carried out amongst several managers. There is no close supervision because each manager is responsible for many people; therefore, communication is easy and occurs directly between members of the organization. For example, a large operating department might have several managers, such as a directorate manager, business manager and clinical manager, and several coordinators or team leaders. The business and clinical managers may be on the same or similar levels, facilitating discussions and meetings on equal terms. Similarly, several team leaders may find that it is easier to discuss problems and opportunities with other team leaders who are in the same position as themselves. However, the flat structure also has several disadvantages. For example, it is more difficult to supervise individuals closely because there is a broad span of control – and there may be confusion if a person has more than one 'boss'. There is also less opportunity for one individual to excel because responsibilities are shared between several people. There is, consequently, more of a need for ongoing education.

The inherent disadvantages of each of these structures have led organizations to look for other structures such as matrix (where a second structure overlays the primary structure) and parallel (where the structure of the department is not linked to the structure of the larger organization) structures. The reality is usually that organizations develop organically in response to the internal and external pressures exerted on them, and they adopt structures that most closely align them to their goals. There is little doubt, however, that some organizations fail to respond to these pressures, and in such cases, there is often employee unrest and problems with output, efficiency and effectiveness.

Organizational functions

An organization functions according to its aims and goals. The functions are usually set out in documents such as philosophy statements, job descriptions, policies and procedures. What the organization achieved in previous years is reported in an annual report; what it intends to do in the future may be described in a strategic plan. In combination, these documents, or others like them, set out what the organization 'does'.

The philosophy or mission statement usually sets out in broad terms the purpose of the organization. It states the beliefs and values that are basic to its operation and may include a list of goals or objectives. Mission statements are often criticized as being too vague or not having substance. However, the real value of a mission statement is the way it guides the overall approach to work within the organization. A mission statement within an operating department may state the core values that its members hold, and the way that the department treats its staff and its patients. Often the mission statement says what the organization is going to do, how it is going to do it and who it is going to do it to.

Job descriptions help to define the organizational structure and function by defining the responsibilities of each individual or position in the organization. Job descriptions tend not to give a complete description of the post-holder's role, but encompass in a wider sense what the individual needs to do to fulfil his or her obligations. In this way, the job can be made flexible to allow for changes and developments. Job descriptions are a key way of controlling individuals within an organization to ensure that each individual contributes to the overall organizational objectives.

Policies and procedures are official statements that guide the behaviour of individuals within the organization. In most cases, they are required by law and by accrediting institutions. For example, the regulatory bodies (Health Professions Council and Nursing and Midwifery Council amongst others) and Quality Assurance Agency regularly review organizational policies to ensure that they help healthcare practitioners to achieve the requirements for registration. Policies exist at every level of an organization from high-level policies relating to overall organizational functions to very specific departmental policies relating to patient care and working practices. The policy manuals of most hospitals are very comprehensive and detailed. They will usually have been written over a period of time in response to situations where decisions had to be made.

The policy manual, therefore, acts as a legal safeguard for the organization or department by establishing standards for practice and quality control. The best policies are evidence based, reviewed regularly, written with input from the people who do the job and written clearly and comprehensively.

Formal communication within an organization is usually enhanced through the use of committees and meetings. The main purpose of committees and meetings is to assist in information gathering and decision making. Their aims are normally to perform a task that cannot be carried out by individuals alone.

Advantages of committees include disseminating ideas and information, coordinating projects and activities, deterring hasty decision making, coordinating actions and broadening individual viewpoints. However, committees often get bad press because of their disadvantages, which can include, for example, difficulty in achieving the action required, excessive time consumption, lengthy discussions, subversion of aims by strong-minded individuals and lack of output. In my experience, the best committees are formed when its members have an inherent desire to achieve their goals. When the need for action is imperative, through urgency or short timescales, then often committees work at their best. When aims are loose or woolly, or the timescales for action are lengthy, the committee meetings can last forever and be unproductive – there is nothing more demoralizing!

While committees are often regulated, formalized and form an important part of the organizational structure, meetings tend to be less formal and often temporary or occur once only. Meetings have three general functions: informational, advisory and problem solving. Meetings need to be structured to work properly, so decisions need to be made beforehand about the purpose of the meeting, who is going to lead it and how the meeting is going to be conducted. While people often disparage committees and meetings for the length of time they take and the possible poor outcomes, meetings and committees are nevertheless two of the most important and powerful tools in the manager's toolkit to help them to perform their functions and roles.

The informal organization

While the formal structure forms the machinery that makes the organization work, the informal structure often oils the bearings to make it work better – or applies the brakes to stop it changing its pace or direction. The informal organization arises to meet the social and interpersonal needs of the members of an organization. The informal organization allows people to negotiate shortcuts to what otherwise might be an onerous process. For example, a company representative who wants to see a consultant surgeon at work might bypass the usual appointment system if he or she develops a good relationship that allows him or her to speak to the surgeon directly. Or a manager might allow a practitioner to finish early one day in return for staying late another. The informal system is very important to ensure the smooth working of the organization, improving communication, preserving the organizations values and for encouraging leaders to develop.

However, as can be anticipated, there are also problems with the informal organization. It can work against the formal organization's rules. For example, the wearing of cover gowns has, for years, been a bone of contention in some areas. A policy that states that cover gowns must be worn while outside the operating department, or that surgical attire must be changed on return to the operating department, can be easily flouted if people 'turn a blind eye' in the interests of speed or convenience. While this is a simple example, such flouting of official policies can, if unchecked, be a major risk to an area's integrity. The informal system might also support resistance to change (Burnes 2004), may turn 'newcomers' into 'outsiders' and may lead to rumours and misinformation through the 'pipelines' or 'grapevine'. The operating department manager must, therefore, be part of the informal organization in order to be able to manage situations such as these. Entry to the informal system is usually through developing interpersonal relationships and a manager who can do this effectively has a great advantage over the manager who cannot form effective relationships with their subordinates. Chapter 12 discusses informal culture further.

Conclusions

This chapter has skimmed the surface of the role of the operating department manager within the greater organization. Untouched are subjects such as budgetary management, risk management, information systems, quality assurance and audit. Some of these topics are covered in the other chapters in this book; other topics can be found in the wealth of books relating to management.

What is clear is that the operating department manager holds a key position in the hospital. The operating department is a challenging environment that provides a baptism of fire for junior managers. However, the skills and knowledge learned in this environment have been proven through experience to prepare people for managing at all levels of a hospital structure. The unique environment of the operating department offers the opportunity to solve problems related to staffing, clinical emergencies, managing large budgets, risk assessment and all the other challenges that managers have to face, deal with and learn from.

Operating department managers of the future will have new challenges to contend with as the internal and external pressure s on the organization change (Ch. 4). For example, the demography of the UK is changing, with an increasing number of elderly. Public expectations of safety and quality of care continue to grow, while the government expects ever greater efficiency and value for money. Much surgery is slowly but surely moving out into the community as people expect treatment closer to their own homes. The roles of staff within the operating department continue to change and grow in response to the increasing specialization of surgery and anaesthesia.

The art and science of management is partly learned and partly inherent. The managers who make a difference will be those who can recognize the potential for change and can capitalize on it, have a vision for the future and can develop a good team of people to carry out their department's activities.

REFERENCES

Bate, P. (2002). The impact of organizational culture on approaches to organizational problem solving. In Salaman G. (ed.) *Decision Making for Business*, Ch. 12. London: Sage.

Burnes, B. (2004). *Managing Change*, 4th edn. Harlow: Prentice Hall.

Hatch, M. (1997). *Organisation Theory*. London: Oxford University Press.

Koontz H. & Weihrich H. (1990). *Essentials of Management*, 5th edn. London: McGraw-Hill.

Meeker, M. & Rothrock, J. (1991). *Alexander's Care of the Patient in Surgery*, 9th edn. London: Mosby.

Mintzberg, H. (1973). *The Nature of Managerial Work*. London: Harper Row.

Mintzberg, H., Ahistrand, B. & Lampel, J. (1998). *Strategy Safari: A Guided Tour Through the Wilds of Strategic Management*. London: Prentice Hall.

NHS Education Scotland (2008). *60 Years of the NHS*. Edinburgh: NHS Education Scotland; http://www.60yearsofnhsscotland.co.uk/history/public-health-challenges/health-improvement/ (accessed 26 October 2008).

Scott, C. & Jaffe, D. (1989). *Managing Organisational Change*. London: Kogan Page.

Sullivan, E.J. & Decker, P.J. (1988). *Effective Management in Nursing*. San Francisco, CA: Addison-Wesley.

Thinkexist (2008). Abraham Maslow Quotes. http://thinkexist.com/quotation/a_first-rate_soup_is_more_creative_than_a_second/222472.html (accessed 16 October 2008).

Whittington, R. (1993). *What is Strategy: And Does it Matter?* London: Routledge.

Williams, C.E. & Tse, E.C.Y. (1995). The relationship between strategy and entrepreneurship: the US restaurant sector. *International Journal of Contemporary Hospitality Management*, **7**, 22–26.

FURTHER READING

Cooke, C. & Slack, N. (1991). *Making Management Decisions*. London: Prentice Hall.

Henry, J. (2001). *Creativity and Perception in Management*. London: Sage/Open University.

Jackson, S. (1998). Organisational effectiveness within National Health Service (NHS) Trusts. *International Journal of Health Care Quality Assurance*, **11**, 216–221.

Lynch, R. (2006). *Corporate Strategy*, 4th edn. London: Pearson Education.

Mano-Negrin, R. & Sheaffer, Z. (2004). Are women 'cooler' than men during crises? Exploring gender differences in perceiving organisational crisis preparedness. *Women in Management Review*, **19**, 109–122.

Schön, D.A. (1991). *The Reflective Practitioner: How Professionals Think in Action*, 2nd edn. Aldershot, UK: Arena.

Strauss, A., Schatzman, L., Ehrlich, D., Bucher, R. & Sabshin, M. (2002). The hospital and its negotiated order. In Salaman, G. (ed.) *Decision Making for Business*, Ch. 7. London: Sage.

3

Action learning: a new way of problem solving in perioperative settings

Anne Jones and Trish Prescott

Key Learning Points

- Provide an understanding of the concept of action learning
- Explore the role of an action learning set and its potential as a continuing professional development experience within perioperative settings
- Examine the potential for action learning as a problem-solving process in the context of a dynamic NHS

Introduction

In 2000 the *NHS Plan* was launched (Department of Health 2000a). Current frameworks for the design and delivery of responsive services are built on the principle of ensuring that clear national standards are developed that are supported by evidence-based guidance. This is in order that the quality of care provided by healthcare professionals is raised (Department of Health 2000b).

In addition, the government is committed to putting quality at the forefront of the NHS: healthcare professionals have a key part to play in this. Quality assurance or health governance requires an inclusive approach embracing all those working within it inclusive of patients and carers. The aim is that clinical practice is evidence based and that best practice is disseminated throughout the service.

Within the *NHS Plan* there was a commitment to ensuring that the NHS should be a model employer (Department of Health 2000a). The provision of

lifelong learning opportunities was seen as fundamental to this. A framework for lifelong learning was developed (Department of Health 2001), which outlined a programme for modernizing learning and development. This was underpinned by the 'Skills Escalator', which is a strategy for recruiting a more diverse range of people to the NHS and for enabling new and existing staff to develop their skills continuously and take on new roles.

In addition to these national directives, the context of practice is enhanced by initiatives to create more flexible working environments, develop more family-friendly policies and address issues related to violence, equality and diversity in the workplace. A significant change was brought about by the introduction of the new national framework for pay, *Agenda for Change* (Department of Health 2003). Within *The Knowledge and Skills Framework* of *Agenda for Change*, NHS jobs were evaluated against a national job evaluation framework with rewards for knowledge and skills as opposed to rewards for time served. In essence, this should provide incentives for staff to take on new responsibilities, change old and existing patterns of working and create new roles that cross boundaries. Given the dynamic nature of change in the NHS, staff members are challenged to change old and existing patterns of working.

The *NHS Plan* (Department of Health 2000a) set the vision for the NHS for the twenty-first century in a 10 year strategy. The Department of Health

Core Topics in Operating Department Practice: Leadership and Management, ed. Brian Smith, Paul Rawling, Paul Wicker and Chris Jones. Published by Cambridge University Press. © Cambridge University Press 2010.

(2008a) *High Quality Care for All: NHS Next Stage Review Final Report* represents the 'next stage' of the reform journey and provides the infrastructure. This document is underpinned by the belief that change should be led within and for the local community by clinicians. This provides opportunities for health-care practitioners to work in partnership, to redesign services and to develop innovative solutions to meet the needs of a patient-focused NHS. The document *A High Quality Workforce: NHS Next Stage Review* (Department of Health 2008b) recognizes that to enable the reforms articulated in *High Quality Care for All* there needs to be corresponding changes to the planning, education and training of the health-care workforce. The document emphasizes the importance of team-based integrated approaches, with clinicians operating as 'practitioner, partner and leader' (Department of Health 2008b:9).

The challenge presented is to subscribe to life-long learning and, subsequently, to enhance and improve the quality of service and care. Illes (2006) would argue that, as healthcare profession-als, they have a body of professional knowledge and practice they need to maintain. In addition, they are in a position to see themselves as possessing positive characteristics of professionalism and have a valuable self-belief.

In setting the context for lifelong learning and continuing professional development, this chapter is focused on action learning as a method of prob-lem solving and learning in groups, in order to bring about change for individuals, teams and their respective organizations in the context of a dynamic NHS. The chapter is grounded in the belief that action learning as a strategy is particu-larly pertinent to the education and development of healthcare professionals, who face unique and often complex practice issues requiring new ways of thinking and partnership working.

Action learning: Where does it come from?

In order to contextualize the action learning approach and its application to the NHS, it is useful to revisit its beginnings. The first reference to what has since become known as action learning was by Revans in 1982. He traced the origins of action learning back to a report about the future of the British Coalmining Industry written in 1945. In this report was the recommendation that a staff college was set up for the industry. The proposal was that in the college the field managers would be encour-aged to learn with and from each other. This would be by their use of a group-review strategy in order to find solutions to the immediate problems that required action – those issues about which some-thing needed to be done. The report specifically said that the college ought not to have any perman-ent staff of experts or lecturers. However, there was no objection to them being invited in for particular missions, after clarity of purpose had been estab-lished. The Mining Association did not go ahead with the proposal, since the coalmining industry was nationalized. It was some years before the National Coal Board did set up its own staff college and partly implemented the first recommenda-tions. Action learning, in the meantime, took on another form, with small groups of managers out in the coalfields working together upon their own and each other's operational problems: deployment of men at the start of every shift, when the mean absenteeism rate might be as high as 15%; main-tenance of new and unfamiliar machinery; ration-alization of supply systems, particularly for timber and other roof supports with escalating costs of all raw materials; and improvement of underground transport systems, which previously utilized the labour of boys and ponies.

This followed the changes after the Second World War and there were no experts with responsibility for running a real pit to send out from headquarters to tell the actual managers how to solve their prob-lems. The men whose task it was to get the coal up the shafts of the pits met at their places of work and discussed what they saw there, making practical suggestions that would then be tried out before the next visit.

During three years of this learning from and with each other, they wrote their own handbook on how to run a coalmine. This was largely done by listing questions they had learned to ask themselves when faced with a unique and perplexing situation. It was the beginning of action learning: to ask, as is inevitable in a world changing as rapidly as ours is today in healthcare, how those responsible for getting things done decide what are the questions to ask themselves when all around seems uncertain and confused and when some of what is sensed within themselves is lack of knowledge and anxiety. Revans (1982) reminds us of the maxim that, when we are in an epoch of change, tomorrow is necessarily different from today, so new things need to be done.

What is action learning?

Pedler (1996) describes action learning as a method of problem solving and learning in groups to bring about change for individuals, teams and organizations. He further supports this by explaining that action learning works to build relationships that help any organization to improve existing operations and to learn and innovate for the future. From this perspective, the key features of action learning are threefold: it is a process rather than a one-off event; it is a form of group learning; and it leads to change.

Weinstein (1999) stresses that there are two other important elements to action learning. These are that it involves a group of people who work together in their learning and that it requires regular and rigorous meetings of the group in order to allow space and time for the questioning, understanding and reflecting on experience at work. Weinstein (1999) goes on to argue that the result of this group learning is the gaining of insights and considerations of how to act in the future. Central to the process of action learning, is the key role of experience. Group members are required to articulate their respective experiences and share them with each other within an environment of learning known as the action learning set (ALS) meeting.

McGill & Beaty (1995:21) support this in their definition of action learning, which is: 'The continuous process of learning and reflection supported by set members, with the intention of getting things done. Through action learning, individuals learn with and from each other, by working on real problems and reflecting on their own experiences.'

> ### Reflective points
>
> - In most of the literature on the subject of action learning, great emphasis is placed on its 'democratic' nature where each individual's input is valued.
> - What would you consider to be the challenges of adopting action learning in your practice area?

Action learning: a framework

A useful framework to underpin action learning has been provided by Krystyna Weinstein (1999:9), who refers to the 'Four P's of Action Learning'.

Examining Programmed Knowledge'. Each individual brings with them knowledge from formal and informal study and experience values, beliefs and assumptions. In ALS, this knowledge is explored and questioned in order to uncover what you already know and what you need to know.

Adhering to the Procedure'. Action learning is a structured approach to learning and it is important that the procedure is followed because this differentiates an action-learning approach from other forms of group problem solving. The procedures involves identification of the project/issue, the ground rules, dedicated time spent discussing issues, active listening and participation and the role of the set, the individual and the facilitator.

Valuing the Philosophy'. Action learning operates in a particular ethos: one of peer support and challenge, active participation, trust, respect, a non-judgemental approach and the creation of a positive enquiring environment for learning.

'*Achieving Two End-Products*'. The output of an ALS has two elements, knowledge and learning: the knowledge gained through working through the chosen problem or issue and the knowledge gained through listening and questioning the experiences of the other set members. In addition there is an output related to a valuable insight in learning to learn and an understanding of how you learn best.

Reflective points

- Considering your practice area, its culture, structure, communication and relationships; what do you feel are the strengths and challenges of introducing action learning?
- Do the strengths outweigh the challenges?

How does action learning work?

Lawson *et al.* (1997) consider the action-learning process in the work organization and believe that for it to succeed in a work context the organization should value the questioning approach on which action learning is firmly based. They argue that the organization's culture should be one where personal development is respected and where employees are trusted with a fair amount of autonomy and that ownership of a problem or task helps in getting things done. The corollary to this then is that line managers need to support their staff for the duration of an ALS project. One of the main contributions of action learning is the creation of a culture of questioning and enquiry.

In an ALS, the issues that are brought to the meeting involve tasks or projects that the group are working on. Revans (1998) refers to these as *problems*, making a useful distinction between what he calls puzzles and problems. He argues that there is, eventually, a known answer when dealing with puzzles. However, he goes on to say that complex issues are faced when dealing with problems which present challenges and opportunities where there may, in fact, be no single solution. Again, a key feature of action learning is option appraisal, leading to the questioning of various ideas and assumptions and gaining fresh insights through this process upon which to base decisions in advance of change.

Weinstein (1999) emphasizes that there is no teaching on what she terms a classic action learning programme. She highlights this as significant as it is probably the most difficult aspects of action learning for participants to understand. Weinstein (1999) argues that action learning builds on experience and prior knowledge. In that light, by sharing information through discussion, the group comes to realize that they have insights and answers of their own, for which they do not need experts to tell them. In the early days of the development of action learning in the coalmining industry, there were no experts to advise those managers.

Reflective points

- Can you think of any problems in your operating theatre which might benefit from this approach?
- Can you see any obstacles to working in this way?
- How do think your colleagues would react to this approach to learning?

Why use action learning?

The answer to why action learning should be used is summarized below:

- it lends itself to complex problem solving, critical levels of reflection, action planning and change
- it is based on a belief in the resourcefulness of the individual
- through its use, individuals learn with and through each other (McGill & Beaty 1995)
- it allows complex problems to be addressed by working and learning together rather than by working in isolation
- it is based on experience and experience is a rich source of learning.

The process of action learning may be new to you and may possibly take longer to explain than to do.

However Pedler (1996) proposes that the best way to understand and appreciate this innovative way of learning, is to experience it personally, and that it is its very simplicity which makes it difficult to explain (Revans 1997).

How does action learning differ from other types of group learning?

Action learning differs from other approaches to group learning because it requires a clear structure to underpin the process and because the issues explored are drawn from the individuals' own experiences. In, for example, problem-based learning, working on case studies or self-help groups, scenarios are developed using the experience of others as triggers for exploration and learning. In the ALS, the group focus is on real work-based issues derived from the direct experience of each individual (McGill & Beaty 1995). Action learning is grounded in the reality of practice and the solutions that are discovered will make a difference to practice. The other important distinction is that the group meetings are only half of the process (Bourner *et al.* 2000). The action-learning approach requires that learning also takes place in practice by taking forward the action agreed at the ALS. Revans (1998:14) is clear that 'there can be no action without learning and no learning without action'.

The structure of action learning

Action learning is based around a small group of people known as the ALS. Meetings follow a format and have a clear purpose, which is to support the discovery of solutions to questions for which there are no simple answers or solutions (Weinstein 1999, Marsh & Wood 2001).

Ideally an ALS has between five and eight members: too small a group will restrict the free flow of ideas while if the group is too large individuals will not be able to spend sufficient time discussing their particular issue in any depth. Where possible, the set should be drawn from individuals who have different perspectives to offer. The ALS approach thrives where there is diversity. Homogeneous sets drawn exclusively from one discipline or one small area may offer a narrow approach to problem solving (Bourner & Frost 1996).

Reflective points

- Consider your area of practice, how many disciplines are represented within the theatre environment?
- List problems from your experience that impact on practice and cross boundaries and individual disciplines.

How often do action learning sets meet?

The frequency of ALS meetings is determined by the reason the group was set up. If they are being used for academic purposes, then the time will be dictated by the length of semesters or module spans. If an ALS is used for personal and professional development, they may run over a 6 or 12 month period, or even longer. If the ALS is based around a particular project, then the time span will reflect this. In all cases, meetings need to be held regularly but allow sufficient time between them for participants to take their agreed action away to follow through prior to feedback at the next set meeting. The length of each meeting will reflect the needs and availability of the group. To allow sufficient time for feedback and the presentation of new issues, set meetings are usually held over a half or a full day.

The set operates by enquiry, reflecting back the issue. Careful questioning allows the presenter of the issue or problem to frame and reframe (Glaze 2002) the problem, exploring different perspectives and gaining new insights. So what at first appears to be the issue may actually be something else after questioning and action. McGill & Beaty (1995:34) suggest that there are three specific stages in the clarification of the issue:

Stage 1: identification of the problem
Stage 2: identification of possible actions
Stage 3: identification of specific action.

Through the process of questioning, an intractable, seemingly messy, indeterminate problem within professional practice gradually takes on shape and clarity and can be viewed through different reflective lenses (Brookfield 1995).

How do meetings work?

An ALS is usually helped to get started through the support of an adviser or set facilitator. The advisor or facilitator encourages the individuals in the group to share ideas and concerns with each other and facilitates the development of the set as a powerful learning system.

If an ALS is made up of people who are experienced in this learning technique, set members can decide whether to incorporate a facilitator role or to self-facilitate. If the group decides to self-facilitate, then they must decide how the roles of the facilitator are to be shared amongst the group. If the ALS approach is new to you or your organization, then it is likely that a facilitated set will be the most productive. Action learning is exactly as it sounds – action and learning – and, correspondingly, the facilitator role is also exactly as it sounds: to enable and empower. Facilitating is not telling or being judgemental, it is allowing others to come to their own decisions about their own issues by creating a positive learning environment (Johnson 1998).

There are specific elements of the ALS approach for which the facilitator takes responsibility. The facilitator's role is to collate the ground rules and to ensure that they are being adhered to, and to oversee that every set member is given an equal chance to discuss and have their chosen topic heard. In the early stages of an ALS, the facilitator may operate in a slightly more directional way, leading the questioning, keeping set members to time, reminding set members to ask open questions and refrain from 'telling' and giving advice. The aim of the facilitator is to scaffold learning and to move the set along a continuum from dependence to independence, and eventually to fade into the background (Vygotsky 1978; cited by Holton &

Clarke 2006). Sets that run over an extended time frame may move naturally from being facilitated to being self-facilitated.

Reflective points

- Is the ALS process anything more than a team meeting of the operating department staff?
- If so, what do you think action learning can offer that differentiates it from other meetings?
- Who might facilitate the ALS and why?

The facilitator does not bring their own issues to the group and this allows them to focus all their energies on the set.

The structured approach of ALS means that every ALS is required to negotiate and agree ground rules. These are fundamental to the effective working of the set and need to encompass and reflect the ethos of the set. Ground rules are individual but the list below represents some common areas to consider:
- confidentiality
- signing up to the ALS framework
- respect
- trust
- keeping an open mind
- active listening to each set member as they present their issue or problem
- giving time to listen and understand their issues
- active participation in each set
- commitment to action between set meetings
- one person to speak at a time
- set members to offer support *and* challenge
- constructive open questions
- keeping a learning contract
- commitment to regular attendance
- mobile phones off or on silent for emergencies
- where, how often and how long to meet for
- flexibility in timing if a set member has a particularly urgent issue or there is little to report on.

This should be used as an initial checklist and then consideration given to adding ground rules specific to the needs of the particular group.

Confidentiality

The set functions in an atmosphere of collegial relationships, trust and safety. Set members need to feel that they can discuss problems of real importance and share with others issues that they do not have all the answers to, without worrying where this information may surface. As a set, members need to decide precisely what they mean by confidentiality. For example, consider whether you would prefer everything discussed to remain confidential? Would you be happy if set members raise general, non-specific details outside of the set? Can projects be discussed if the individuals and organizations are not named? Would it be appropriate for individual set members to discuss with others what they have learned through ALS? This takes some time to discuss and agree, but it is important and needs to be in place before the set begins to operate. If the set is being used in professional practice and individuals are bound by codes of professional conduct, then this needs to be understood and clearly stated in the ground rules.

The facilitator can also decide when it might be appropriate to employ other problem-solving techniques if they feel that the set is struggling to progress an issue and is becoming stalled. Strategies can include fishbowl exercises, where for a limited time the presenter of the issue sits outside of the set and listens to the discussion but does not participate. This can act as a useful catalyst when a set becomes stalled. Alternatively, a SWOT analysis (strengths, weaknesses, opportunity, threats) (Pickton & Wright 1998), force field analysis (Lewin 1951), mind mapping or an exercise to identify circles of influence and concern (Covey 1992) may be required to unlock a particularly difficult issue.

The role of the set member

The role of the set member has two elements. The first is to bring issues to the group, to commit to taking action after each set meeting, to feed back the results of the action and to be open to new ideas. The second element is to be part of the 'listening mirror' (Weinstein 1999:57). This requires active, focused listening when other set members are presenting their issues. In other groups, it may be possible to opt out, or 'tune out' of discussions and choose what you pay attention to. However, in an ALS, the expectation is that the set member will give (and receive in return) their full attention. Each set member will also learn from listening to how others tackle their problems and will be able to transfer this vicarious learning into their own workplace. The process may feel strange at first and it is unusual for an individual to be afforded the opportunity to focus on an issue for a period of time, but you will quickly get used to this different and rewarding way of working.

The set is not there to give advice but to provide support and challenge in equal measure. The facilitator aims to achieve a balance between a benign atmosphere that does not stretch its members and, at the other extreme, a competitive, interrogatory environment where set members are reluctant to speak.

The set functions by shedding reflective light through questioning, so that the presenter is enabled to understand and focus on their issue or area of concern and is empowered to progress an action plan of their choosing in order to address or resolve their concern (McGill & Beaty 1995). Questions asked by set members need to be pertinent and asked where there is a genuine desire to discover the answer. Challenging questions may be uncomfortable but they are constructive and are designed to prompt the closer examination of assumptions and beliefs. Some examples are:

- How does that make you feel?
- What else could you do?
- What do you want out of this situation?
- What are your options?
- What is the worst thing that could happen?
- Why do you think that is?
- What is the issue?

Set members need to be able to give time and space to the individual presenting their issue, to accept silences and to hear not only what is being said but what is left unsaid. McGill & Beaty (1995) offer a useful analogy for ALS meetings, likening them to episodes in a series, because the issues presented are the threads which link each meeting. The reviews of progress on action at the beginning of the session are the highlights and the new issues raised are the content of this week's episode. Action learning in this way is concerned with reflection and learning from past experience, but it is also future orientated because of the focus on action and change.

Action learning: the outcome

Engagement with action learning develops a range of valuable transferable skills. In addition to the new knowledge and understanding gained from working on issues and projects of your own and others, the ALS member gains an insight into how one learns. Action learning provides an opportunity to be exposed to other ways of working and provides a conceptual bridge that enables awareness of other perspectives to develop. It also develops an appreciation of partnership and cross-boundary working and learning; enhances communication, active listening and discriminatory questioning skills; and encourages the use of problem-solving techniques, critical thinking and critical levels of reflection. Being part of an ALS can also develop empathy, peer support, self-awareness, time and project management skills and the ability to accept and respond positively to challenging questioning.

Conclusions

This chapter has provided an outline of the origins of action learning, which has been presented as a process of learning within a group, using real work issues and firmly based on the experiences of the group members. In order to distinguish action learning from other ways of learning in groups, a distinction was made between the ALS and other group-learning activities such as problem-based learning, working on case studies or self-help groups, to name three examples.

A theoretical framework for action learning has been offered (Weinstein 1999). The infrastructure for the action-learning approach has been explained in defining the role of the facilitator and the set members. This illustrated the process and provided a practical guide for the reader.

In this chapter, clarification of the key elements of action learning has been provided for those who have a general interest, prior knowledge or previous experience. For the reader for whom this chapter has been an introduction to the concept of action learning, the concluding comments are in agreement with Pedler (1996) and his suggestion that the best way to understand and appreciate this innovative way of learning is to experience it for yourself.

REFERENCES

Bourner, T. & Frost, P. (1996). The experience of action learning in higher education. *Education and Training*, **3898**, 22–31.

Bourner, T., Cooper, A. & France, L. (2000). Action learning across a university community. *Innovations in Education and Training International*, **37**, 2–9.

Brookfield, S.D. (1995). *Becoming a Critically Reflective Teacher*. San Francisco: Jossey-Bass.

Covey, S. (1992). *The Seven Habits of Highly Effective People: Personal Workbook*. London: Simon Schuster.

Department of Health (2000a). *The NHS Plan: A Plan for Investment, a Plan for Reform*. London: The Stationery Office.

Department of Health (2000b). *A Health Service of all the Talents: Developing the NHS Workforce*. London: The Stationery Office.

Department of Health (2001). *Working Together: Learning Together. A Framework for Lifelong Learning for the NHS*. London: The Stationery Office.

Department of Health (2003). *Agenda for Change: Modernising the NHS Pay System*. London: The Stationery Office.

Department of Health (2008a). *High Quality Care for All: NHS Next Stage Review Final Report*. London: The Stationery Office.

Department of Health (2008b). *A High Quality Workforce: NHS Next Stage Review*. London: The Stationery Office.

Glaze, J.E. (2002). Stages in coming to terms with reflection: student advance nurse practitioners' perceptions of their reflective journeys. *Journal of Advanced Nursing*, **37**, 265–272.

Holton, D. & Clarke, D. (2006). Scaffolding and metacognition. *International Journal of Mathematical Education in Science and Technology*, **37**, 127–143.

Illes, V. (2006). *Really Managing Health Care*, 2nd edn. Milton Keynes, UK: Open University Press.

Johnson, C. (1998). The essential principles of action learning. *Journal of Workplace Learning*, **10**, 296–300.

Lawson, J., Beaty, L., Bourner, T. & O'Hara, S. (1997). Action learning comes of age – part 4: where and when? *Education Training*, **39**, 225–229.

Lewin, K. (1951). *Field Theory in Social Science*, New York: Harper Row.

Marsh, P. & Wood, B. (2001). Pressed for results – an action learning project in practice. *Industrial and Commercial Training*, **33**, 32–36.

McGill, I. & Beaty, L. (1995). *Action Learning in Practice*. London: Kogan Page.

Pedler, M. (1996). *Action Learning for Managers*. London: Lemos & Crane.

Pickton, D.W. & Wright, S. (1998). What's SWOT in strategic analysis? *Strategic Change*, **7**, 101–109.

Revans, R.W. (1982). *The Origins and Growth of Action Learning*. Bromley, UK: Chartwell Bratt.

Revans, R.W. (1997). Action learning: its origins and nature. In Pedler, M. (ed.) *Action Learning in Practice*, 3rd edn, pp. 3–13. Aldershot, UK: Gower.

Revans, R.W. (1998). *The ABC of Action Learning: Empowering Managers to Act and to Learn from Actions*, 2nd edn. London: Lemos & Crane.

Vygotsky, L.S. (1978). *Mind in Society: The Development of Higher Mental Processes*. Cambridge, MA: Harvard University Press.

Weinstein, K. (1999). *Action Learning: A Practical Guide*, 2nd edn. Aldershot, UK: Gower.

4

Agenda for change: what do theatre staff need to know?

Joy O'Neill

Key Learning Points
- Understand the genesis of the recent remuneration strategies in the NHS
- Appreciate the underpinnings of the *Agenda for Change* approach to pay settlement
- Identify the elements of a grade determination under *Agenda for Change*
- Identify special considerations that apply to perioperative staff in setting pay grades

Leadership within the operating theatre is essential to create an environment for staff development and the delivery of effective patient care. Managers have the responsibility to contribute to healthcare planning and the promotion of policy development. The rationale for recent modernization of the health service, to ensure that care provision is of high quality and is supported by the appropriate planning framework, has been set out in strategic health and social policy documents (Department of Health 2000, 2004a).

It is important for managers and other clinical leaders to have a repertoire of skills and interventions that can be used to motivate and engage clinical teams in risk assessment and continuous quality improvement at the level of patient care delivery (Ferguson *et al.* 2007).

Agenda for Change

The *Agenda for Change* (AfC) was introduced as an initiative to modernize pay and grading within the NHS (Department of Health 2004b). This significant change for managers would initiate a new pay structure and terms and conditions for all health-related staff including perioperative practitioners.

In the *NHS Plan* (Department of Health 2000), the government stated its intention to invest in better remuneration for nurses in line with the increased clinical responsibility engendered through the rapid pace of change in healthcare and increasing workload.

The AfC involves a process of negotiation for a much needed pay modernization system for the NHS: a system that will effectively replace the existing clinical grading and local pay arrangements. It will have a massive impact on perioperative staff as discretionary points and on-call and standby allowances will be replaced by the new system (Beesley 2002).

Government proposals in 1999 by the four UK countries highlighted the need for change and, most importantly, for a pay system based on the premise of equal pay for work of equal value.

The introduction of AfC represents a fundamental change to the terms and conditions of the employment of the vast majority of staff employed in the NHS (Health Protection Agency 2003).

All posts subject to AfC were evaluated by a panel of trained personnel (composed of staff and management representatives). In these evaluations, issues considered were job experience, clinical skills and patient care. The factors that carried the most points or weight concerned knowledge, skills

Core Topics in Operating Department Practice: Leadership and Management, ed. Brian Smith, Paul Rawling, Paul Wicker and Chris Jones. Published by Cambridge University Press. © Cambridge University Press 2010.

and experience, reflecting the importance of knowledge in the delivery of NHS care. Members of staff were given a banding based on this evaluation.

The fundamental building block of the new pay system is the job evaluation scheme, which will be used to determine basic pay for all staff in the NHS (Kirwan 2004).

All members of staff receive a knowledge and skills job post outline relating to their banding that contains six core elements and other specific dimensions which identify their roles, experiences and responsibilities. The practitioner's training and development remain central to pay progression.

The Knowledge and Skills Framework

The Knowledge and Skills Framework (KSF) (Department of Health 2004c) and its review process is one of three developments of AfC implementation, the other two being job evaluation and terms and conditions of employment.

The KSF defines and describes the knowledge and skills which NHS staff need to apply in their work in order to deliver quality services (Royal College of Nursing 2006). The KSF has been introduced as part of the AfC reforms in the UK to link pay and career progression to competency (Gould *et al.* 2007).

There are two purposes to the KSF. First, it is a design tool for all staff (excluding medical staff) in the NHS and, second, it is a link to pay progression for the different members of staff within all departments of Trust hospitals. The KSF has been developed as part of the AfC package and has been designed to promote fair opportunities for continuing professional development (CPD), pay and career progression throughout the NHS (Department of Health 2003).

The KSF can introduce changes in practice and improve communication with patients, carers and the multidisciplinary care team. This, in turn, can promote effective patient care, support effective lifelong learning and staff development. It helps to clarify staff roles and responsibilities and to support equality and diversity between all types of staff within a Trust. It can improve skill mix, identify training needs and aid recruitment and retention of staff. It allows the manager to identify governance requirements, clinical training resources and improve workforce planning.

The KSF has wide-ranging implications for all non-medical staff employed in the NHS. Some of the changes that result will be of a positive nature, but others will represent a challenge to practitioners, their managers and to higher education. If KSF operates as intended, training needs will be assessed more accurately and this could have a positive, albeit challenging, influence on educational commissioning, with purchasers able to demand programmes of CPD more appropriate to their needs (Gould *et al.* 2007).

The KSF should also encourage healthcare providers to develop other progressive human resource practices such as effective recruitment, selection, retention, service redesign and the development of new roles (Fletcher & Williams 1985, Borrill *et al.* 2000).

Hospitals employing a higher proportion of well-qualified nurses generate more favourable patient outcomes than those which do not (Aitken & Patrician 2000).

Banding

Each member of staff has a post outline written for their job that describes the roles and responsibilities to be undertaken in that job. Each job has six core elements and other specific dimensions in the post outline. The core elements are communication, personal and people development, health and safety and security, quality and equality and diversity. In addition, there are many different specific dimensions that define other responsibilities in the different roles.

At defined points on each member of staff's pay band, there are two gateways. These are designed to ensure development in the job and, as a result, to reward staff with pay increments. At these gateways, a formal review takes place of the individual's development against the job's full KSF post outline. It is to confirm that individuals are applying their knowledge and skills consistently to meet the full demands of their post.

The *foundation gateway* occurs no later than 12 months after an individual is appointed to a pay band, regardless of the pay point to which the individual is appointed. The purpose of the foundation gateway is to check that individuals can meet the basic demands of their post.

The *second gateway* is at a fixed point towards the top of the pay band. It also allows the reviewer to examine if the practitioner has further developed their skills and fulfils the responsibilities of their role and is at a fixed point before the top of the band. Having an agreed post outline in place is crucial in measuring individual development within a post, thus facilitating continued pay progression. Post outlines are for individual roles, agreed in partnership in individual-employing organizations. As such, there will no doubt be variability to some degree between the post outlines set up by different organizations (Royal College of Nursing 2006).

In the event of inadequate achievement, the reviewer and the practitioner will devise an agreed action plan to address the relevant issues to ensure a successful outcome in the next few months. The reviewer will prioritize the practitioner for development in order to maximize the individual's chances of success in passing through the gateway.

If the department has not been able to meet its responsibilities for supporting development for the practitioner through financial constraints, lack of managerial support as agreed in the previous annual appraisal, limited human resources or lack of learning opportunities in the work place, the practitioner will progress through their gateway and the increment paid.

An appeal can be held if the reviewer or the practitioner is in disagreement with the result of the appraisal. The parties should follow their Trust appeal process.

Appraisals or personal development reviews

An appraisal is an annual process which provides the practitioner with an opportunity for a formal and structured discussion regarding his or her work performance over the previous year. It is a two-way process where it gives the practitioner the opportunity to discuss needs for CPD and progress in his or her present role. It should be conducted in a quiet and supportive environment. It can assist in the planning of performance development for the next year, promote further CPD and support internal and external learning and development.

Traditionally the reviewer and the practitioner agree training needs during the appraisal, which in most Trusts take place annually. However, evidence from the National Audit Commission (2001) has indicated that for many NHS employees, including nurses, no regular assessment of training needs occurred.

With the implementation of AfC, appraisal is obligatory at least once a year and possibly more often if an individual or their manager is not satisfied with progress or performance.

Members of staff have an appraisal or personal development review each year to discuss their development, provide feedback on their progress within their role and assess their learning and development needs through the use of their KSF and post outline. This two-way process is an opportunity for the practitioner to discuss their progress, any concerns, their training needs and receive feedback from their reviewer.

The practitioner produces a portfolio of evidence which will be discussed during the meeting.

The appraisal

The reviewer gives the practitioner a date and time for the appraisal. This is usually three to four weeks prior to the date to allow time for preparation of the portfolio.

The reviewer will pre-book a room and ensure privacy and a quiet environment for the meeting.

The practitioner can ask the reviewer for an informal meeting to discuss the appraisal process. The practitioner can also seek advice on completion of the portfolio from the reviewer or their work colleagues. The reviewer will review the practitioner's portfolio evidence, ensuring that there is sufficient effective evidence to meet the requirements of the core and specific dimensions of the post outline. This meeting gives both parties an opportunity to assess whether the practitioner's performance and development has matched the identified objectives. The discussion should be open and positive, identifying the strengths and weaknesses of the practitioner. Constructive feedback can be given on the previous annual performance. If further evidence is necessary, time can be given to the practitioner to gather further evidence within an agreed timescale.

The practitioner needs to identify any personal learning need objectives for the following year, to be discussed with the reviewer, because, at the end of the meeting, set objectives will be decided and agreed.

National Health Service Careers (2007) identifies the 'smarter criteria' which should be used for the next year's objectives. They describe these criteria as:

specific: describing the desired outcome in as much detail as possible

measurable: identifying what measures will be used to judge whether or not this has been achieved

achievable: reflecting the way the practitioner enjoys learning and with objectives agreed as, the more say the practitioner has in setting the goals, the more likely he or she is to achieve them

realistic: building on personal development opportunities that can be taken up at work

time bound: being those new goals to be completed before next year's appraisal, plus some milestones which might be set to help in monitoring progress

evaluated: seeing how successful the practitioner has been as part of ongoing monitoring, not just in the period immediately before the next appraisal.

The appraisal is an opportunity for the reviewer and the practitioner to have an honest, two-way discussion on the previous and following annual performance. It should be a positive experience for the practitioner and give an opportunity to assess progress and provide future expectations of his or her role.

The portfolio

The CPD standards of the Health Professions Council (HPC) state that operating department practitioners (ODPs) should maintain a continuous, up-to-date and accurate record of their CPD activities (Health Professions Council 2008). From 2008, each time ODPs renew their registration the HPC will ask a random sample of registrants to fill in a CPD profile and return it with evidence of how they have met the standards (Health Professions Council 2008). This means that the first audits for ODPs will occur in 2008. If selected for audit, the ODP will have to provide evidence of CPD for their previous two years of practice (Health Professions Council 2008).

Nurses as part of their post-registration education and practice requirements for the Nursing Midwifery Council (NMC) need to maintain a personal profile. The purpose of this is to record their learning activity for re-registration purposes. A profile is a personal document. It has two functions. It contributes to registrants' professional development by helping them to recognize and appreciate their abilities, achievements and experiences. It also provides an information source that registrants can refer to in order to collect material about standards of education following registration (Nursing Midwifery Council 2008).

Both ODPs and nurses need to produce a portfolio for their annual appraisal to provide relevant evidence for the core and the identified specific dimensions in their post outline and the competences of their job. This portfolio can also be used for the HPC and NMC if required at annual re-registration.

Each core and specific dimension has four levels, with a description of how knowledge and skills need to be applied at that level. Evidence collected needs to correlate with the specific dimension that the practitioner's post outline identifies.

Layout of the portfolio is optional but it could include personal details, curriculum vitae, post outline, objectives, mandatory lectures' record and evidence.

The evidence will identify training and development within the job on a day-to-day basis. The reviewer will be aware of the candidate's experience and will have observed their practice. The evidence could be verbal, observational, hand-written or electronic and include reflective accounts within the candidate's practice.

Evidence can include a previous annual appraisal record, any CPD records, patient documentation, adverse incidents, work colleagues' testimonies, mandatory lecture attendance and reflective accounts.

Reflection is a systematic enquiry into one's own practice to improve practice and deepen understanding in order to assist in the assessment of career objectives, the analysis and value of daily experiences, the development of an ownership of practice and an appreciation of patient care, and to allow a change, if necessary, in practice.

Reflection evidence can include critical incident analysis, reflective accounts of practice, an audit of practice and an account of strengths, weaknesses, opportunities and threats (SWOT).

Use of e-learning and information technology

NHS Elite has published a booklet for each of five of the six core dimensions at each of the four levels.

All the KSF dimensions are mapped to relevant associated national occupational standards (National Health Service ELITE, 2008).

Similarly, other companies provide information for KSF e-learning.

Teamwork

Effective teamwork between practitioners in the operating theatre can ensure the delivery of efficient patient care by perioperative nurses and ODPs.

Sigurdson (2001), states that the operating room as a functional context relies on effective multi-disciplinary teamwork, which makes the operating theatre such a dynamic and challenging area in which to work.

The multiprofessional and disciplinary team of surgeons, anaesthetists, nurses and ODPs all work together to ensure that the individual patient's perioperative journey is as comfortable as possible. Communication needs to be effective between all the members of the team during the pre-, intra- and postoperative care of the patient. The Kennedy Report (Department of Health 2001: Ch. 22, p. 2) decribed this as follows: 'Teamwork is of crucial importance . . . collaboration between professionals is at the core of what we mean by teamwork . . . teamwork as a means of serving the patient implies a multiprofessional team and a sharing of responsibility. . . teamwork is the collaborative effort of all those concerned with the care of the patient'. Leggat (2007) believes that, although effective teamwork has been consistently identified as a requirement for enhanced clinical outcomes in the provision of healthcare, there is limited knowledge of what makes health professionals effective team members and even less information on how to develop skills for teamwork.

Teamwork is essential in the provision of healthcare. The division of labour among medical, nursing and allied health practitioners means that no single professional can deliver an episode of healthcare (Sicotte et al. 2007).

Surgery depends on interprofessional teamwork, which is becoming increasingly specialized. If surgery is to become a highly reliable system, it must adapt and professionals must learn from and share tested models of interprofessional teamwork (Healey *et al.* 2006).

REFERENCES

Aitken, L.H. & Patrician, P.A. (2000). Measuring organisational traits of hospitals: the revised nursing work index. *Nursing Research*, **49**, 1–8.

Beesley, J. (2002). Making sense of the agenda for change. *British Journal of Perioperative Nursing*, **12**, 177–182.

Borrill, C., West, M.A., Shapiro, D. & Rees, A. (2000). Teamwork and effectiveness in health care. *British Journal of Health Care*, **6**, 364–371.

Department of Health (2000). *The National Health Service (NHS) Plan*. London: The Stationery Office.

Department of Health (2001). *Final Report: Learning from Bristol: The Report of the Public Enquiry into Children's Heart Surgery at the Bristol Royal Infirmary [CM 5207]*. London: Stationery Office.

Department of Health (2003). *The NHS Knowledge and Skills Framework (NHS KSF) and Development Review Guidance: Working Draft*. London: The Stationery Office.

Department of Health (2004a). *The National Health Service (NHS) Improvement Plan; Putting People at the Heart of Public Services*. London: The Stationery Office.

Department of Health (2004b). *Agenda for Change*. London: The Stationery Office.

Department of Health (2004c). *The NHS Knowledge and Skills Framework (NHS KSF) and the Development Review Process*. London: The Stationery Office.

Ferguson, L., Calvert, J., Davie, M. & Fallon, M. (2007). Clinical leadership: using observations of care to focus risk management and quality improvement activities in the clinical setting. *Contemporary Nurse; A Journal for the Australian Nursing Profession*, **24**, 213–225.

Fletcher, C. & Williams, R. (1985). *Performance Appraisal and Career Development*. London: Hutchison.

Gould, D., Berridge, E.J. & Kelly, D. (2007). The National Health Service Knowledge & Skills Framework and its implications for continuing professional development in nursing. *Nursing Education*, **27**, 26–34.

Healey, A.N., Undre, S. & Vincent, C.A. (2006). Defining the technical skills of teamwork in surgery. *Quality & Safety in Health Care*, **15**, 231–234.

Health Professions Council (2008). *Your Guide to Our Standards for Continuing Professional Development*. London: Health Professions Council.

Health Protection Agency (2003). *Human Resources and Remuneration Committee. Enclosure 03/58*. http://www.hpa.org.uk/web/HPAwebFile/HPAweb_C1194947366552.

Kirwan, G. (2004). Agenda for Change. *Emergency Nurse*, **12**, 16–17.

Leggat, S.G. (2007). Effective healthcare teams require effective team members; defining team competencies. *BMC Health Services Research*, **7**, 7–17.

National Audit Commission (2001). *Hidden Talents. Education and Training for Healthcare Staff in NHS Trusts*. London: Audit Commission.

National Health Service Careers (2007). *Me and my PDR; A Workbook for Personal Development Review*. London: NHS Careers, NHSLD01.

National Health Service Elite (2008). *eLearning, IT Essentials and the Knowledge & Skills Framework. NHS Connecting for Health. Education & Training & Development*. London: NHS Elite.

Nursing Midwifery Council (2008). *The PREP Handbook*. London: Nursing Midwifery Council.

Royal College of Nursing (2006). *Guidance for RCN Members on the NHS Knowledge & Skills Framework*. London: Royal College of Nursing.

Sicotte, C., Pineault, R. & Lambert, J. (1993). Medical interdependence as a determinant of use of clinical resources. *Health Services Research*, **28**, 599–621.

Sigurdson, H. (2001). The meaning of being a perioperative nurse. American operating registered nurse. *AORN Journal*, **74**, 205; **78**, 213–217.

5

The SWOT analysis: its place in strategic planning in a modern operating department

Julie Smith

Key Learning Points

- Develop an understanding of the SWOT (strengths/weaknesses/opportunities/threats) analysis
- Discuss how SWOT can improve on perioperative service delivery
- Develop skills in objectively analysing the clinical environment

Introduction

Since the UK Government White Paper (Griffiths, 1984) on reforming the NHS and the introduction of NHS Trust hospital status; the NHS has become a business driven by productivity and income generation. Services beyond the operating department have also been affected; in particular general practitioners (GPs) face a more challenging workload of treating patients and managing busy practices. Like GPs, hospital managers have also been charged with the responsibility and accountability of managing financial budgets for their department/services. While these changes to health policies strengthen the management of patient services and managerial autonomy, they do not come free from tensions among healthcare staff. Change management in the NHS since the late 1970s has become a key aspect of a manager's role. It has been argued the NHS is in a constant state of 'flux' and changes to staff roles are viewed as a threat, leading to resistance to change and dissatisfaction.

Any business wishing to succeed in a constant changing world needs to be ready and agile enough to respond to new demands. This perhaps is what the NHS has achieved since the mid 1970s in response to new health demographics.

Many practitioners will have been involved in past changes and probably recognize the terms 'just-in-time' management, 'quality circles' and so on. While personal experiences of those management techniques may be mixed, adopting and evaluating their application can help managers to cope with, and maximize their responses to, strategic change. In this chapter, the term strategic change is used to denote change that has an impact on the whole department, for example implementing a new infection control policy or practice.

The SWOT analysis is one particular tool that has been adopted and is in frequent use in healthcare practice. In simple terms, SWOT analyses the strengths, weakness, opportunities and threats associated with strategic change.

The SWOT tool has been used by many businesses since the 1970s, many of which have found the tool to be invaluable in maintaining an advantage over their competitors. Their diligent application of the tool offers opportunities for analysis and decision making to ensure the correct change that is for the greater good of the organization.

In healthcare, it can be applied in the same way to ensure the greater good for the patient as well as the organization's aims and objectives. This has

Core Topics in Operating Department Practice: Leadership and Management, ed. Brian Smith, Paul Rawling, Paul Wicker and Chris Jones. Published by Cambridge University Press. © Cambridge University Press 2010.

been the case in many operating departments, where more investment has been made in technology and buildings to keep up with the demands of the public. Operating department staff continue to work in an environment where changing technology, increased targets and productivity place a high degree of pressure on their professional abilities. Therefore, it is no surprise that operating department practice has been likened to Henry Ford's production of motor vehicles: the factory production line. Although parallels may be drawn with commercial businesses, such as that of Henry Ford, the distinct difference for perioperative practitioners is the focus on vulnerable patients.

Whatever change practitioners introduce to their working practices they must ensure that they uphold a 'duty of care' to the patient by providing a high-quality service based on robust sources of evidence. To achieve this, practitioners must develop an awareness of their environment and how they can contribute to such excellence in care. In a modern health service, this approach will encourage increased numbers of expert patients who are fully informed about their treatment, leading to a true patient-led service (NHS Plan; Department of Health 2000).

Application of the SWOT tool can help practitioners to achieve this by meticulously considering and appraising the areas of concern, identifying aspects for improvement and addressing elements of practice in a way that can improve service delivery.

At the time of writing, many practitioners will be part of hospitals applying for Foundation Trust status, where the hospitals can govern their own activities. Given the increased responsibility and accountability of being a Foundation Trust holder, then perioperative practitioners will also be charged with ensuring that what they offer their patients is timely and appropriate. Consequently, adopting the SWOT tool in the operating department can allow managers to analyse their practices continuously, such as list management, staffing, mentoring and identify the weak areas. This might be useful in identifying future staff training on new equipment or might assist with change in policies.

Irrespective of what arises, the one advantage of staff engagement is empowerment among the 'shop-floor' workers to make informed decisions on how the operating department can provide a quality service and an enjoyable career as a perioperative practitioner.

What is SWOT?

SWOT is an acronym of strengths, weakness, opportunities and threats. It is a tool for challenging and considering all factors relating to the topic under question. It is also useful for team building and is often taught or used on management courses. Although it is well known, it is worth considering further how simple and effective it can be.

SWOT is a simple, systematic method that can be adopted by staff at all levels. It was originally presented in Switzerland in 1964 by Urick and Orr (Chartered Institute of Personnel and Development 2008), who in the 1970s shared the concept in the UK with commercial companies such as WH Smith and Sons. The tool continues to be at the heart of the success of many commercial companies.

Albert Humphrey (Business Balls 2004), one of the 'founding fathers' of SWOT, commented,

This approach captures the collective agreement and commitment of those who will ultimately have to do the work of meeting or exceeding the objectives finally set. It permits the team leader to define and develop coordinated, goal directed actions, which underpin the overall agreed objectives between levels of the business hierarchy.

SWOT is easy to use, simple to present and very cost-effective. Many practitioners prefer SWOT because of its simplicity of use in a grid formation (Fig. 5.1).

To complete the boxes in Fig. 5.1, the rule of thumb among team discussions is to keep the questions simple. Ask the questions and note the answers that arise by filling in the grid. This will help to reveal the specific details that are required to lead to a strategic change.

Strengths	Weaknesses
Opportunities	Threats

Figure 5.1 A simple SWOT grid.

Use of SWOT enables proactive thinking rather than habitual or instinctive reactions; therefore, it encourages broader thinking. Encouraging practitioners to dissect an idea or aspect of the work environment enables them to highlight areas of concern or weakness. This method is particularly useful in analysing and improving traditional theatre rituals, many of which are grounded in culture and the 'way things are done around here'. The SWOT analysis helps to modify these practices by applying advances in technology and the evidence base.

Example of SWOT: the operating suite orthopaedic education week

This project by the South Eastern Sydney Illawarra Area Health Service was entered in the Baxter 2006 NSW Health Awards, Education and Training category.

'The restructure of South Eastern Sydney and Illawarra Area Health Services resulted in transference of elective orthopaedic services from the St. George Hospital to the Sutherland Hospital. To assist in the transfer of services, an education program based around orthopaedic surgery was developed by the Nurse Educator of the Operating Suite. A SWOT analysis and an analysis of the program stakeholders were performed to determine the viability of the program. A needs assessment was utilized to identify the unit's education deficits and this was transferred into

---

the program specifics. The program was implemented after a tasks analysis and a transfer of learning framework had been completed. Post course evaluations showed positive feedback from the participants and it was deemed to be successful and a valuable program for the Hospital.'

http://www.archi.net.au/elibrary/health_administration/ awards06/ed_training/op_theatres

---

Examples of SWOT analysis in action

In the example below, a team is looking at why theatre lists failed to begin on time. Figure 5.2 shows use of the SWOT grid to examine problems with the supply of orthopaedic prostheses.

Strengths

As it suggests, the strengths assessment identifies strengths such as resources, knowledge, assets and levels of productivity. The strengths of the team would be identified as:

- human resources: theatre team on duty, on time to begin the list
- resources available to operate on patients
- porter available to collect patient
- patient on ward
- surgeon and anaesthetist available on time to begin theatre list
- operating list compiled previous day, with correct patient details and surgical procedure
- correct documentation and equipment available to enable the patient to be sent for
- good communication between ward and operating theatre staff.

Weaknesses

The second part of the analysis would observe problems (weaknesses) in the system or 'chinks in the armour', that is, reasons for failure to start operating on time:

- staff late for duty: sickness or absence
- resources unavailable: instrument sets not sterile through packaging damage; loan sets late

Strengths	Weaknesses
A variety of orthopaedic prosthesis available	Reordering and delivery of prosthesis can be delayed
Readily available	Some sizes may remain on the shelf
Opportunities	**Threats**
Micro-management of stock	Overstocking may cause lack of funding for other theatre consumables

Figure 5.2 Example of use of the SWOT grid to examine the supply of orthopaedic prostheses.

arriving; problems in sterile services department such as loss of steam, volume of activity, and reduction in staffing

- too few porters to cope with demand: recruitment or sickness absence issues
- patient not arrived: no bed available on ward; patient not prepared for theatre; preoperative clinic malfunction such as blood tests or electrocardiography not performed or not available
- surgeon or anaesthetist late in arriving
- incorrect details on operating list, such as wrong ward or patient details
- inadequate system to get patients to theatre such as send slips not available (needing printing out), insufficient trolleys (e.g. too many out for repair) or insufficient canvas sheets (laundry issue)
- poor communication between ward, surgeon and anaesthetist.

Opportunities

The opportunities assessment looks for potential areas for improvement and development; using the areas highlighted in the strengths and weaknesses, such opportunities can be developed:

- operate a strict policy for punctuality, ensuring all staff are aware of the importance of beginning on time; manage sickness and absence policy
- ensure resources available on the previous evening, ordering loan equipment in adequate time for arrival, checking and sterilization; liaise with sterile services department regularly

- make a business case for more porters; stagger send times for each theatre, thus ensuring porter's availability; manage sickness and absence policy
- encourage liaison with ward, the previous night if possible, regarding patient problems and change the order of the list if required
- encourage punctuality of surgeons and anaesthetists; ensure the theatre is ready for list start time, highlighting problems with doctors; record late start of list and reason
- checklist prior to start time for correct details; have amendments typed up and change all lists
- ensure all documentation and resources required to send for the patient and transport to theatre are available at beginning of day and in full working order; have equipment repaired as soon as possible after reported broken
- encourage communication between all members of the disciplinary team.

Threats

External influences that may prevent components of the analysis being achieved are listed as threats:

- staff failing to adhere to policy; long-term absence; overtime bill increased as staff cover other staff
- sterile service department having maintenance problems, causing delays in equipment: joint venture
- lack of finance to employ more staff: resource management
- operating lists inadequate (avoid by compiling these the previous night)
- poor communication between staff on wards and theatre; failure to pass on information between shifts
- doctors repeatedly late in starting; list management impossible; patients at risk of having their procedures cancelled; breach dates can occur or sessions removed
- funding unavailable for repairs (deal with by capital bid for replacement equipment); time factor increased with reduced equipment.

Conclusions

The SWOT analysis is not a sophisticated tool that needs detailed training on how to use it. It was designed (Chartered Institute of Personnel and Development 2008) to offer a guided exploration of an aspect of business or commerce, and now health practice, which might need to undergo some change. Simple but informed questioning of practice assists staff at all levels to contribute and take ownership of the strengths, weaknesses, opportunities and threats and make recommendations to their employer based on their findings. The grid diagram used in SWOT is simply a representative picture of the debate that might take place among operating department staff when challenged to find a solution or a strategic approach to yet another change in their clinical practice. Although this has been a brief overview of SWOT, the best way to appreciate the value of the tool is by applying it in practice.

REFERENCES

Business Balls (2008). *SWOT analysis*; http://www.businessballs.com/swotanalysisfreetemplate.htm (accessed 22 August 2008).

Chartered Institute of Personnel and Development (2008). *SWOT analysis*; http://www.cipd.co.uk/subjects/corpstrtgy/general/swot-analysis.htm (accessed 22 August 2008).

Department of Health (2000). *The NHS Plan: A Plan for Investment, a Plan for Reform*. London: The Stationery Office.

Griffiths, R (1984). *Report, NHS Management Inquiry Report*. London: The Stationery Office.

6

Corporate governance: setting the scene for perioperative practice

Claire Campbell

Key Learning Points
- Appreciate the nature of corporate governance
- Understand the public policy initiatives that gave rise to corporate governance in healthcare
- Appreciate the implications of failing corporate governance

Introduction

Corporate governance is the way in which governing boards direct, control and manage organizations and public bodies. One of the roles of stakeholders is to recognize an organization's obligations to society. Good governance leads to good management, performance and financial management, and ultimately to good outcomes for patients and organizations.

This chapter will identify the core principles of good governance, the underlying corporate governance codes, their application and the roles and responsibilities of all involved. The aim of good governance is to understand accountability for the benefit of all stakeholders, including patients.

Adopting a comprehensive corporate governance framework is the cornerstone of sound business conduct and is fundamental to the success of an organization. Failure in governance is a threat to the future of organizations. This was seen in recent examples of poor corporate governance in healthcare, for example in the organ retention scandals,

and in business, for example the events at Enron and Maidstone (discussed later in this chapter).

Healthcare bodies in the UK and worldwide subscribe to corporate governance codes; consequently, organizations and those who work within them should challenge substandard governance. The information provided in this chapter will focus on information about the NHS in England, although NHS Scotland and Wales use similar if not identical principles.

NHS boards run within an integrated governance context but also need to run within the broader governance perspective. This is particularly true when considering legal frameworks as described by Monitor (the Independent Regulator for NHS Foundation Trusts), which bring a more commercial approach to regulation within the NHS (Department of Health 2006).

The Organisation for Economic Co-operation and Development (2004:11) defines corporate governance as 'a set of relationships between a company management, its board, shareholders and other stakeholders . . . providing the structure through which the objectives are set and the means of attaining those objectives and monitoring performance'.

In this context the 'company' can be seen as the organization. 'Shareholders' normally hold shares in private companies. However, members of organizations or Foundation Trusts could also

Core Topics in Operating Department Practice: Leadership and Management, ed. Brian Smith, Paul Rawling, Paul Wicker and Chris Jones. Published by Cambridge University Press. © Cambridge University Press 2010.

be seen as shareholders because of the role they play in supporting the organization. Finally 'stakeholders' within the health context include staff, patients, the local population, voluntary and charity organizations related to health and patient groups.

The Audit Commission (2003:4) offers a more succinct definition for corporate governance: 'The framework of accountability to users, stakeholders and the wider community, within which organizations take decisions, and lead and control their functions, to achieve their objectives'.

So, why is this relevant? Everyone works in an organization, whether in a permanent or agency role and, therefore, understanding and appreciation of corporate governance will enable each person to challenge poor or substandard governance within their organization.

These principles can refer to places of work, such as healthcare establishments, but also nursing, perioperative, education or management organizations, for example the Association for Perioperative Practice or the College of Operating Department Practitioners.

Reflective point

- What is the relevance of corporate governance to your healthcare system, your organization and you as an individual?

Corporate governance in the United Kingdom

In the UK, corporate governance considers principles of good practice that encompass common law and political contexts. A desire for more transparency and accountability has stimulated the introduction and development of corporate governance. High-profile financial and corporate scandals have also driven NHS Trusts to implement corporate governance.

Corporate governance has not developed in a vacuum but has arisen because of a series of investigations that have taken place in the UK over recent years (Jones & Pollitt 2003).

The following reports and guidance have been developed by committees appointed by government departments and include support or leadership from respected individuals from business and industry, who have given their name to the final report. They are overviewed by Jones & Pollitt (2003).

The Cadbury Report in 1992 identifies board responsibilities in financial reporting. It outlines expected behaviours within business and public life to ensure good practice in governance. This includes the setting up of governing boards, and the reporting and control mechanisms.

The Greenbury Report (1995) recommends principles on director's salary. This includes setting up remuneration committees containing non-executive directors and full disclosure of the individual remuneration package. The NHS has carried out these recommendations and they are readily seen in the annual reports of hospitals and Primary Care Trusts and independent healthcare providers. The Hempel Report (1998) reviews the Cadbury and Greenbury Committee recommendations and approves the findings of the precursor reports.

The Higgs Review (2003) contains many recommendations, including the structure of the board, the role and other commitments of the chair, the role of the non-executive director, the recruitment and appointment procedures to the board and the induction and professional development of directors, including board tenure and time commitment.

The Smith Review (2003) highlights the importance and clarified the role of audit committees, particularly about the need to ensure systems of control are in place but not to undertake the monitoring themselves.

The Combined Code (1998) drew together the recommendations of Cadbury, Greenbury and Hempel in its original publication and was updated in 2003 (Combined Code 2003) to include guidance from both the Higgs and Smith Reviews and it represents best practice for UK companies.

International governance

Healthcare bodies in the UK and Europe subscribe to corporate governance reform particularly within public health. All countries subscribe to voluntary, non-binding principles of corporate governance and have resisted taking an enforced approach within healthcare and business systems. Comparisons of European companies show some to have obligatory guidance and some to have recommendations or non-binding guidance.

Following the passing of the Sarbanes–Oxley (SOX) Act in 2002 in the USA, regulatory and legally enforceable corporate governance rules were introduced that detailed criminal and civil penalties for non-compliance; these became effective in 2006. This Act came into being because of the US corporate financial scandals involving Enron and WorldCom.

UK health organizations undertaking joint enterprises, or where partner organizations have US connections, need to consider the SOX Act 2002 (Department of Health 2006).

The principles of public life

As well as subscribing to the principles of corporate governance considered above, most NHS boards are also required to uphold the 'seven principles of public life' from the Nolan Committee (1995). They are not statutory but apply to all aspects of public life and were set up by the Nolan Committee for the benefit of all those who serve the public in any way from ministerial or UK Government level to NHS Trust boards and organizations. Over the years, many bodies have adopted them or their own versions of them. The seven principles are:

selflessness: requires holders of office to take decisions solely for public interest, not to gain financial or material benefits for themselves, family or friends

integrity: requires holders of office not to place themselves under any financial or other obligation to individuals or organizations that might influence their performance of their duties

objectivity: requires that individuals make decisions or choices solely on merit

accountability: requires decision makers to be accountable for their decisions and actions

openness: requires holders of office to be as open as possible, only restricting information when the wider public interest clearly demands this, for example during tender applications or when disclosing patient information

honesty: requires holders of office to declare any private interests about their public duties, for example declaration of interests of speakers at conferences

leadership: requires holders of office to promote and support these principles by leadership and example.

Reflective point

- How do these seven principles apply to you in everyday working?

Codes of conduct

The *National Health Service Code of Conduct for NHS Managers* (Department of Health 2002) complies with the Nolan principles. All NHS bodies have to take all reasonable steps to comply with this managerial code. This clearly applies to the NHS, under its title, although the Department of Health states that it also applies to independent healthcare units providing services to the NHS and to NHS staff managed by them (Shifrin 2002).

This code has two purposes; it provides guidance for managers in the decisions and choices they make, and it reassures the public that managers make these decisions against a background of accountability and professional standards.

The managerial code of conduct was implemented as a response to the Bristol Royal Infirmary

Inquiry Final Report (Department of Health 2001a), known as the Kennedy Report.

Reflective points

- Review the Code of Conduct for NHS Managers and your professional code of conduct (if applicable).
- How do these compare with the Nolan principles: are there common characteristics?

Principles of good governance

There is much information published that identifies principles of good governance in the NHS and other public bodies. This includes, for example, the following documents:

- *Corporate Governance, Improvement and Trust in Local Public Services* (Audit Commission 2003)
- *Governing the NHS, A Guide for NHS Boards* (NHS Appointments Commission 2003)
- *Building Effective Boards* (Barker 2004)
- *Good Governance Standard for Public Services* (CIPFA, JRF & OPM 2005)
- *NHS Audit Committee Handbook* (Department of Health 2005)
- *NHS Foundation Trust Code of Governance* (Monitor 2006)
- *Integrated Governance Handbook* (Department of Health 2006)
- *The Intelligent Board* (2006)
- *The Intelligent Commissioning Board* (2006).

The following section reviews several of these documents, to help to identify common themes that support good governance.

Corporate Governance, Improvement and Trust in Local Public Services (Audit Commission 2003) suggests that good governance combines 'hard' factors – systems and processes – and 'soft' factors – leadership and behaviour – and integrates the following internal and external environmental factors:

- visionary leadership
- open and honest culture

- systems and processes that support accountability, for example internal controls with reliable and robust supporting information
- consideration of external diverse opinions.

The document also offers six core principles of good governance. It states that good governance means:

- focusing on organizational purpose and outcomes
- performing effectively in clearly defined roles
- promoting values for the organization and displaying these values through behaviour
- taking informed, transparent decisions and managing risk
- developing the capacity and means of the governing body to be effective
- engaging stakeholders with genuine accountability.

Governing the NHS, A Guide for NHS Boards (NHS Appointments Commission 2003) identifies the roles of the board, chair and chief executive and outlines the governance framework as containing:

- strategic planning and objective setting
- ensuring clinical, risk and finance procedures support achievement of the objectives
- ensuring ways of working demonstrate satisfactory controls.

Building Effective Boards (Barker 2004) identifies three features that high-performing boards require:

- the structures and roles of the organization and the board and the relationships between the board, the organization and key stakeholders are clear and fit for purpose
- the actions and behaviours of the board and its key stakeholders work in the best interest of the public to deliver outcomes
- the organization uses objective and constructive performance evaluation to ensure performance improvements.

The principles contained within the *Good Governance Standard for Public Services* (CIPFA, JRF & OPM 2005) build on Nolan by setting out six core principles of good governance for public service organizations. These principles aim to encourage organizations, departments and individuals to review their own effectiveness, providing common principles for assessing good governance practice and providing a basis for both staff and the public to challenge substandard governance (CIPFA, JRF & OPM 2005). This document states that good governance:

- focuses on the organization's purpose and on outcomes for citizens and service users
- performs effectively in clearly defined roles
- promotes values for the whole organization and displays the values of good governance through behaviour
- takes informed, transparent decisions and manages risk
- develops the ability of the governing body to be effective
- engages stakeholders and makes accountability 'real'.

The *Integrated Governance Handbook* (Department of Health 2006) identifies the following key principles for boards to deliver good governance:

- clarity of purpose
- a strategic annual agenda
- an integrated assurance system in place
- intelligent information to support decisions
- review and simplification of committee structures, with clear terms of reference
- strengthening of the audit committee
- appointing board support, for example the company secretary role
- selection, development and review of board members
- agreed board etiquette
- development of individual board members.

The *Intelligent Board* (2006) focuses on the information required by the boards of Acute Trusts to perform their work. It identifies the need for those charged with governing NHS organizations to have access to high-quality, timely information. This would, in turn, enable the board to set the strategic direction, manage progress towards strategic goals and monitor performance.

These documents contain several themes which are overriding and commonly stated in good governance. The organization should have:

- clearly defined organizational purpose, strategic direction and objectives

- clearly defined work, roles and responsibilities of individuals and groups (e.g. committees)
- informed, transparent and collective decision making
- decision making supported by robust, reliable, 'intelligent' information
- capacity and capability development of the individuals charged with governance
- regular reviews of board and individual performance
- clearly stated values of the organization that are displayed through behaviour
- effective stakeholder engagement
- good leadership
- internal and external controls in place that support accountability
- board assurance of major organizational risks, financial performance
- a strategic annual agenda cycle in place.

Warning signs of service failure

How can managers recognize substandard governance? The analysis of public inquiries has identified common themes which have been developed into the seven generic warning signs of service failure:

1. Poor leadership
2. Low levels of accountability
3. Failure to address known problems in working relationships
4. Insular organizational culture with poor customer focus or community engagement
5. Poor strategic risk management
6. Lack of clarity of roles, responsibilities and accountabilities within and between organizations
7. Poor decisions based on inadequate information.

If leaders do not set an effective tone and culture for the organization, a 'club culture' can prosper, which can result in small influential power bases within which climates of fear, misinformation, malpractice and lack of supportive governance systems can flourish.

Poor working relations can lead to a 'toxic' working environment with communication between professional groups breaking down and hierarchies hindering effective team or multidisciplinary working.

A closed culture can lead to an internal focus with weak or hostile relations with external agencies and lack of appreciation or adoption of good practice. This, in turn, can also lead to failure to engage users and the public, leading to a lack of understanding of community concerns.

A lack of clarity can lead to poor staff and performance management practice, poor supervision and performance, a lack of current policies and inadequate staffing as an outcome.

Poor information for decision makers can result in organizations failing to recognize the impact of policy decisions, failing to challenge information, accepting information at face value and accepting outdated information (Audit Commission 2003).

The section below on examples of poor governance outlines how ignoring these warning signs can result in disastrous results for end-users (patients) and the organization.

Challenging standards of governance

Several of the documents listed above under 'Principles of good governance' offer self-assessment tools to monitor, review and challenge an organization's governance.

By asking the following questions, operating department managers can test their department's or organization's governance and identify areas for development.

Purpose and outcomes:
- What does your department/organization do; what is it for?
- Is there a clear explanation of what your department/organization is doing?
- How widely known are the department/organization's aims and objectives, both internally and externally?

- What is the quality of perioperative and organizational services provided?
- What is being done to improve perioperative/organizational services?
- How does the department/organization spend its money?
- Does the department/organization show any of the signs of organizational failure, as outlined by the warning signs of service failure?

Roles, responsibilities and functions:
- Who is in charge?
- How are they appointed (or elected)?
- Who is responsible for what at departmental/board level?

Organizational values:
- What are the department/organization's values?
- Are the values followed in practice?
- What standards of behaviour should be expected?
- Are the Nolan principles put into practice?
- What is the culture of the department/organization?

Decision making and management of risk:
- Who is responsible for which decisions in the department/organization?
- What decisions have been taken and how were they made?
- Are decisions based on robust, timely information and guidance?
- What risks are there to the department/organization? How are these communicated?
- Who is the department/organization accountable to and for what?

Leadership:
- Are there clear support systems in place for staff development?
- Is there an appraisal system in place?
- Are independent staff surveys carried out to show how effective are the two-way communication, information and management systems in place?

Engagement:
- Are there opportunities for people (staff and stakeholders) to make their views known?
- Are there opportunities to get involved and is this encouraged?

- What support is available for people who do get involved?
- Are decisions made because of opinions being asked for and listened to?
- Does the department/organization provide opportunities to question the leadership about plans and decisions?
- Is there a clear complaints process and procedures to respond to suggestions in place?
- Does the organization publish an annual report containing accounts and other information about the organization's progress against objectives? Is the content made interesting and is it freely available?
- Are answers to all these questions easily obtained?

Corporate governance is the brain and nervous system of the organization; when it is working well, this provides clear direction, anticipation of danger and good communication, movement and action, while receiving information to enable remedial action and changes of course if required.

> Reflective point
>
> - What systems are in place within your organization that are underpinned by good governance?

Examples of poor governance

So why should managers carry out corporate governance? Is it of value to an organization? Poor governance can result in a poor experience for service users, such as failures in care because of poor understanding or appreciation of the organization's values. There have been many examples of inquiries in the health service and commercial business in recent years because of poor governance. Three examples are given below.

Organ retention inquiries

Three major organ retention inquiries have been held so far in the UK: Alder Hey (Department of Health 2001b), Bristol (Department of Health 2001a) and more recently the Isaacs Report (Department of Health 2003). These inquiries identified the following governance issues:

- failures to involve patient's families
- a lack of informed consent and medical ignorance of the considerations of religious or cultural beliefs
- a lack of insight, openness and honesty by medical and other hospital staff
- lack of leadership and teamwork with an imbalance of power
- lack of internal reviews of quality, resulting in continuing poor mortality rates
- concerns when raised were not taken seriously
- lack of independent external monitoring to review patterns of performance over time and to identify good and failing performance.

The organ retention inquiries stemmed from the long-standing and widespread practice of removal and retention of organs following post-mortem examination. The lack of consent for these procedures and the unlawful practices carried out were contrary to the rules of the Human Tissues Act 1961 (cited by Chief Medical Officer 2001).

Because of these inquiries, a new Human Tissues Act (2004) was passed and the Human Tissue Authority was set up to regulate the removal, storage, use and disposal of human bodies, organs and tissues. The Human Tissue Authority is responsible for giving advice and guidance on the Human Tissue Act 2004. It has issued codes of practice to give practical guidance and lay down the standards expected by those carrying out activities which lie within its remit.

Enron

The collapse of Enron in 2001 started a chain of events resulting in the identification of financial irregularities within other leading corporations and a later sequence of major bankruptcies in the USA. The outcome of this was the passing of the SOX Act 2002 in the USA.

The Enron company resulted from the merger of two Houston pipeline companies, which then diversified into a trading company for the energy industry and later plastics, metal and telecommunications. The company had a reputation publicly as a model company, with the executives enjoying close working relations with the highest level of politics in the USA and supported by reported high earnings. The media reported the company's success positively to the business community and added to the organization's competitive culture. Before declaring bankruptcy in 2001, the energy trading firm was the seventh largest company in the USA. The following examples of poor governance led to the demise of Enron:

- failure to disclose financial irregularities, and fraudulent reporting on the balance sheet
- lack of transparency, which misled investors, creditors and market regulators and prevented them having a clear understanding of the financial standing of the company
- systematic conflicts of interest, which enabled bending of rules for organizational and personal gain; this included conflicts among the chief financial officer and other senior officers of the company and role confusion and overlap between the external auditor and the management
- a leadership and organizational culture actively cultivated by the president and chief executive officer that was independent, innovative and aggressive, with unchecked ambition, 'stretching' of rules and an erosion of ethical boundaries
- failure of the moral and ethical boundaries of decision making, with resulting deception and exploitation of investors and customers
- absence of internal controls
- poor, inaccurate and misleading board information.

The collapse of Enron resulted in thousands of people losing their jobs, savings and pensions. Criminal proceedings found Kenneth Lay, Chief Executive Officer, and Jeffrey Skilling, President and Chief Operating Officer, guilty of 25 of 34 charges of conspiracy and fraud in 2006. This followed four years of investigation by the US Department of Justice's Enron Task Force. Many other Enron executives have subsequently been convicted in court cases across the USA (Sims & Brinkmann 2003, Clarke 2004).

Outbreaks of *Clostridium difficile* infection

The Healthcare Commission (2007) investigated outbreaks of *Clostridium difficile* infection at Maidstone and Tunbridge Wells NHS Trust. Section 52(1) of the Health and Social Care (Community Health and Standards) Act 2003 empowers the Healthcare Commission to conduct investigations into healthcare provided by or for an English NHS body. The Commission investigates when allegations of serious failings are raised, chiefly when these include concerns of patient safety. The Healthcare Commission's findings raised many examples of poor governance:

- lack of attendance at various governance and risk committees, with these committees not providing acceptable leadership and support to the directorates
- the system intended to highlight clinical risks to the board did not work effectively and the board were not aware of issues and problems faced at ward level
- confusion over accountability because of several changes to the governance structures and responsibilities within the organization
- the board rarely considering or resolving matters requiring strategic input as a board or within the committees with authority delegated by the board
- no robust systems in place to follow up actions required or consider lessons learnt
- the chief executive controlled board information and there were delays in reporting information and following actions required; information was incomplete and inaccurate about the outbreaks, which resulted in the board not carrying out its accountability to the public effectively
- new board members were not provided with effective induction on their assurance role or

basic infection control information, resulting in an inability to study and challenge information, an integral part of the role of a non-executive

- leadership style of the chief executive and the culture of the organization was described as autocratic and reactive, with poor delegation, an unfocused direction and a difficulty to challenge.

Reflective point

- In reviewing each of the examples, which of the seven generic warning signs of service failure can be identified?

Conclusions

Good corporate governance is more than making sure things do not go wrong or fixing them if they do. It adds value and ensures effectiveness in an ever changing environment.

Corporate governance is concerned with both the internal and the external running of an organization, and it offers essential mechanisms that support achieving objectives by contributing performance measurements to sustain progress towards this achievement.

The UK NHS has adopted common core principles following the publishing of several reports; such changes have gained momentum in recent years because of several high-profile governance failures.

Corporate governance is relevant not only to healthcare organizations and their departments or directorates but also to other educational, commercial and professional organizations.

All members of an organization have the responsibility to challenge poor or substandard governance. Governing boards and managers must take final responsibility for the organization's performance, complying with principles of good governance.

Well-governed organizations are well placed to achieve and sustain high-quality services, which will lead, eventually, to improved patient care.

REFERENCES

Audit Commission (2003). *Corporate Governance, Improvement and Trust in Local Public Services.* London: Audit Commission; http://www.auditcommission.gov.uk.

Barker, L. [for HM Treasury Public Services Productivity Panel] (2004). *Building Effective Boards: Enhancing the Effectiveness of Independent Boards in Executive Non-Departmental Bodies.* London: The Stationery Office.

Cadbury, A. (1992). *Report of the Committee on the Financial Aspects of Corporate Governance.* London: Gee.

Chief Medical Officer (2001). *Report of a Census of Organs and Tissues Retained by Pathology Services in England.* London: The Stationery Office.

CIPFA, JRF & OPM (2005). *Good Governance Standard for Public Services.* London: CIPFA, JRF & OPM.

Clarke, T. (ed.) (2004). *Theories of Corporate Governance.* London: Routledge.

Combined Code (1998). *Combined Code, Principles of Corporate Governance.* London: Gee.

Combined Code (2003). *The Combined Code of Corporate Governance.* London: Gee.

Department of Health (2001a). *The Report of the Public Inquiry into Children's Heart Surgery at the Bristol Royal Infirmary 1984–1995: Learning from Bristol [Cm 5207 (II)].* London: The Stationery Office.

Department of Health (2001b). *Royal Liverpool's Children's Inquiry Report.* London: The Stationery Office.

Department of Health (2002). *National Health Service Code of Conduct for NHS Managers.* London: The Stationery Office.

Department of Health (2003). *The Isaacs Report. The Investigation of Events that Followed the Death of Cyril Mark Isaacs.* London: The Stationery Office.

Department of Health (2005). *NHS Audit Committee Handbook.* London: Department of Health and the Healthcare Financial Management Association; http://www.library.nhs.uk/healthmanagement.

Department of Health (2006). *Integrated Governance Handbook. A Handbook for Executives and Non-executives in Healthcare Organisations.* London: The Stationery Office.

Greenbury, R. (1995). *Directors' Remuneration.* London: Gee.

Hempel, R. (1998). *Committee on Corporate Governance: Final Report.* London: Gee.

Health and Social Care (Community Health and Standards) Act 2003; http://www.opsi.gov.uk/acts/acts2003/ukpga_20030043_en_1.

Healthcare Commission (2007). *Investigation into Outbreaks of* Clostridium difficile *at Maidstone and Tunbridge Wells NHS Trust*. London: Healthcare Commission.

Higgs, D. (2003). *Review of the Role and Effectiveness of Non-Executive Directors*. London: Department of Trade and Industry.

Human Tissue Act (2004). Chapter 30; http://www.opsi.gov.uk/acts/acts2004/ukpga_20040030_en_1.

Jones, I. & Pollitt, M. (eds.) (2003). *Working Paper No. 277: Understanding How Issues in Corporate Governance Develop: Cadbury Report to Higgs Review*. Cambridge, UK: ESRC Centre for Business Research, University of Cambridge; www.cbr.cam.ac.uk/pdf/wp277.pdf (accessed 20 April 2009).

Monitor (2006). *The NHS Foundation Trust Code of Governance*. London: Monitor; http://www.monitor-nhsft.gov.uk/home/our-publications/browse-category/guidance-foundation-trusts/mandatory-guidance/code-governance (accessed 20 April 2009).

NHS Appointments Commission (2003). *Governing the NHS, A Guide for NHS Boards*. London: NHS Appointments Commission.

Nolan Committee [Committee on Standards in Public Life] (1995). *First Report into Standards in Public Life*. London: The Stationery Office.

Organisation for Economic Co-operation and Development (2004). *Principles of Corporate Governance*. Paris: OECD.

Sarbanes–Oxley (SOX) Act (2002). US Legislature.

Shifrin, T. (2002). Public Sector is bound by code. *Health Service Journal*, **112**, 6–7.

Sims, R. & Brinkmann, J. (2003). Enron ethics (or culture matters more than codes). *Journal of Business Ethics*, **45**, 243–255.

Smith, R. (2003). *Audit Committees Combined Code Guidance*. London: Financial Reporting Council.

The Intelligent Board (2006). *The Intelligent Board Point 10: The Intelligent Board for Acute Trusts*. London: The Intelligent Board Steering Group; http://www.appointments.org.uk/docs/intelligent_board_report.pdf (accessed 20 April 2009).

The Intelligent Commissioning Board (2006). *The Intelligent Board: Understanding the Information Needs of SHA and PCT Boards*. London: The Intelligent Board Steering Group; http://www.appointments.org.uk/docs/intelligent_board_report.pdf (accessed 20 April 2009).

FURTHER READING

Clarke, T. (ed.) (2004). *Theories of Corporate Governance*. London: Routledge.

Mallin, C. (2004). *Corporate Governance*. New York: Oxford University Press.

McLean, B. & Elkind, P. (2004) *The Smartest Guys in the Room: The Amazing Rise and Scandalous Fall of Enron*. London: Penguin Books.

7

Managing different cultures: adversity and diversity in the perioperative environment

Rita J. Hehir

Key Learning Points

- Importance of managing differing cultural assumptions within an overall culture of theatre practice
- Development of policies in the theatre environment that respect cultural and lifestyle diversity
- Consequences of failing to address bullying and disrespect among the theatre workforce

At the outset in this chapter, it is necessary to point out that much of the literature around some of these topics is generated from research outside the UK and is related to nursing. However, the origins of the material do not mean that it is lacking in relevance or resonance for all perioperative practitioners in the UK. A manager in an operating department, regardless of seniority or length of time in post, has the role of managing that area and in doing so can contribute to the creation of a more productive and healthy workplace environment (Advisory Conciliation Arbitration Service 2008).

Evidence of problems

There is a plethora of legislation to protect all workers in the UK, in particular those who belong to minority groups, and it could be argued that any issues around the management of these groups should have become history a long time ago.

Despite this, it is all too common to hear of the NHS being described as 'institutionally racist' (McPherson 1999). In fact, 'One in five nurses in Scotland has been bullied in the past year' (BBC News 2006:1). Quine (1999) also states that 42% of a sample of British nurses who participated in a study on bullying believed they had been victims of bullying in the previous year.

The phrase 'nurses eating their young' was used by Griffin (2004) to describe disapproving attitudes towards newly qualified nurses, suggesting that there is a culture amongst more senior qualified staff of not being supportive or encouraging towards newly qualified practitioners, who should continue to be taught and sustained.

In 2005, Trevor Phillips, Chair of the Commission for Racial Equality, described the NHS as 'a snow-capped mountain where the boss is almost always white'. The lack of senior executives from ethnic minorities (estimated at just 1% of chief executives and 7% of executive directors) is especially stark when one considers that nearly 35% of doctors, 16% of nurses and 11% of non-medical staff are from ethnic minorities. Esmail (2005) and Giga et al. (2008) both conclude that there is a higher incidence of bullying experienced by black and ethnic minority members in the workplace compared with other members.

Although difficult to quantify, anecdotal evidence gleaned from discussions with students and clinical colleagues suggests that the dominant culture

Core Topics in Operating Department Practice: Leadership and Management, ed. Brian Smith, Paul Rawling, Paul Wicker and Chris Jones. Published by Cambridge University Press. © Cambridge University Press 2010.

within many operating theatre departments is that of 'survival of the fittest'. In keeping with this culture is the suggestion that to be overly sensitive or to expect the most basic respect from your co-workers sets someone apart as not being quite tough enough to function effectively within the perioperative team.

The clarion call can be heard from different generations of perioperative practitioners that in 'our day' the absence of equality laws and 'political correctness gone mad' made for a better working life. The supposition seems to be that valuing and respecting colleagues somehow undermines the quality of the care delivered to patients.

The premise of this chapter is to suggest that there is no contradiction or conflict of principles between managing an effective, productive workforce and creating an environment in which all grades of staff are treated fairly. In addition, I hope to demonstrate that there is no disparity between being responsive to the needs of minority groups within a team and the responsibility as a manager to address individual performance deficits or resort to disciplinary procedures when and if necessary without fear of accusations of bias and prejudice. This principle should apply equally to all staff, including majority groups, disabled persons, ethnic minorities, and those with differences in gender, sexual orientation, religious or health status.

This may seem a tall order and it could be questioned what has it to do with culture and diversity within the perioperative team? Where is the link to patient care, which is our primary goal?

Capable leadership and management in system structures within healthcare are fundamental to the delivery of a positive patient experience (Department of Health 2007). Fortunato (2000) comments: 'The patient is the reason for the existence of the healthcare team. He or she looks to the perioperative team to fulfil his or her diverse needs during the perioperative, intraoperative and postoperative phases of care'.

A useful starting point may be to define the use of the word culture within the context of this chapter. Taking one of the available definitions of culture,

'the customs, civilization and achievements of a particular time or people' (*Concise Oxford Dictionary* 1992:282), frees the discussion from the more frequent and rigid interpretation of culture as referring to the needs of members of ethnic minorities, individuals with alternative lifestyles or those who are not members of the majority faith group.

A restricted interpretation of the word can also suggest that 'cultural differences' is something disconnected from the majority that has to be endured and accommodated in order to avoid getting into difficulty with such concerns as 'the race card/disabled card' or any other 'card' being used against managers when they are required to address legitimate concerns about the work or ability of an individual from a minority group.

Information point

The term 'race card' may be perceived as a derogatory phrase. It is not intended to be offensive in the context of this chapter. The term has its origin in card-playing parlance meaning to play a trump card to gain advantage. It appears in this chapter because it is a common element of the lexicon of management in perioperative settings (*The Phrase Finder* 2008).

Drennan (1992; cited by Brown 1998:3) provides a definition of culture in more accessible terms, describing culture as 'how we do things around here'. It is what is typical of the organization, the habits, the prevailing attitudes and the pattern of accepted and expected behaviour that has grown up.

This, in turn, leads to reflection on the culture of the operating theatre. In each individual department, there is the question of how we do things around here and how we initiate new members of staff into that culture. Is the culture of the theatre suite a positive or a negative one? How does a person work out how to fit in? What are the consequences of being seen as 'different'? To explore some answers, it is interesting to reflect on the following points.

The overall goal of the NHS is to create a culture based on the following principles: a place where all staff, whatever their differences, feel valued and have a fair and equitable quality of working life; where differences between individuals are accepted and where the benefits that diversity brings to the staff, the organization and to patients and clients in particular are valued. Everyone wants to feel part of a workforce that feels valued and confident.

All employees are protected by Equal Opportunity, Race Relations and Human Rights Acts. Many members of staff may also be protected by the Disability Discrimination Act. This comprehensive umbrella of defensive shielding may suggest that the possibility of being a victim of discrimination as an employee is negligible if not downright impossible, yet the material reviewed above provides some evidence that this is not the case.

How is racism, bullying, lateral violence, discrimination and incivility manifested in the workplace?

Lateral violence, which is sometimes referred to as horizontal violence (Patterson 2007), is seen as inappropriate behaviour between members of the same social or professional group: for example, hostility that is nurse to nurse or practitioner to practitioner. It can be visible in the following unprofessional and oppressive behaviours: 'Non-verbal innuendo, verbal affront, undermining activities, withholding information, sabotage, infighting, scapegoating, backstabbing, failure to respect privacy, and broken confidences' (Griffin (2004) cited by Stanley *et al.* 2007). Further actions that may constitute lateral violence and incivility include verbally abusive language; intimidation tactics such as threatening team members with retribution, litigation, violence or job loss; sexual comment; racial slurs and ethnic jokes; shaming or criticizing team members in front of others; and throwing instruments or objects around.

Bullying has been described as offensive behaviour though vindictive, cruel, malicious or humiliating attempts to undermine an individual or group of employees.

The 'silent' treatment is another common expression of bullying behaviour: communicating through a third party, discussing a team member as if they were invisible and criticizing accents, appearance or work performance.

The Health and Safety Executive (2005) defines bullying within its policies on work-related violence as 'any incident in which a person is abused, threatened or assaulted in circumstances related to their work'.

When considering these concepts of oppressive conduct, it would be very difficult to categorically insist that such behaviour is never witnessed in the perioperative environment.

> ### Reflective points
>
> - Are any of these behaviours visible in your workplace? What is your contribution to the culture of your theatre?
> - Do you support patients and colleagues, or do you see no harm in 'having a joke' at their expense even though it might be damaging?

Causes of problems

Tradition is frequently blamed for this culture. The unequal balance of power between medical staff, historically playing a patriarchal role, and nursing staff, occupying a subsidiary role, is considered one of the culprits (Kelly 2006). Lack of resources, increased workload and raised stress levels can contribute to a burgeoning in bullying behaviour (Stevens 2002). Discriminative and oppressive behaviour thrives in poorly managed, unaccommodating working environments where members of staff feel undervalued through the failure to provide chances of continuing learning or career development (Taylor 2004).

In periods of financial restraints, it is not uncommon for these conditions to be found in all areas of the NHS; consequently, it is easy to see why this culture of aggression can become an insidious and unchallenged part of everyday life in the operating theatre.

The consequences of poor working relations

It is important to bear in mind that poor working atmospheres, tension and conflict within a team inevitably lead to the delivery of a poor service to the client (Bolchover & Brady 2004). Bullying can lead to mental health problems and to financial problems for the victim if they are forced to leave work. Discord in the workplace can give rise to poor practice, which has a direct adverse impact on the care patients receive.

Discrimination and bullying play a big part in creating staff shortages as this kind of culture compels its victims to seek alternative employment.

The annihilation of a very valuable and scarce resource is another potential consequence of oppressive behaviour. A study by Hadikin & O'Driscoll (2000) found that over half the midwives interviewed in their investigation of bullying intended to leave the midwifery profession.

In a report commissioned by the International Labour Organization, Hoel *et al.* (2001) estimated that the cost of work-related stress could be in excess of £1.8 billion per year. This figure does not include loss of productivity as this is impossible to assess.

The highest price of bullying is probably that paid by the victim, however, who suffers loss of confidence and self-esteem and is denied the right to work in their chosen career. It is entirely possible that the ultimate cost of oppressive behaviour can be the act of suicide by the victim.

The responsibility of a manager

The responsibility of a manager (at departmental manager level or team leader level l) is to achieve the outcomes set for the department by managing people and resources effectively. It is the manager's job to function with integrity. Managers have to contribute to reaching the targets set for the department and to the overall aims of the entire organization and also will teach, supervise, maintain standards, overcome obstacles, motivate staff and resolve conflicts (Morris 2001).

Templar (2005:xi) specifies the obligations of the manager's role:

you are responsible for a whole gang of people that you probably didn't pick, may not like, might have nothing in common with and who perhaps don't like you very much. You have to coax out of them a decent day's work. You are responsible for their physical, emotional and mental safety and care. You have to make sure that they don't hurt themselves or – each other. You have to ensure that they carry out their jobs according to whatever legislation your industry warrants. You have to know your rights, their rights, the company's rights, the union's rights.

This may seem a tall order taken in the context of running an operating department, with the added responsibility of managing diverse groups of staff as well as ensuring, above all, that the patient receives the best care and treatment. The good news is that there is an endless supply of down-to-earth practical initiatives that can be employed by a manager to eliminate all forms of poor practice in their department. The principal tools available to a manager in an operating department are the Code of Conduct for Nurses (Nursing and Midwifery Council 2008a) and the *Standards of Conduct, Performance and Ethics* for operating department practitioners (Health Professions Council 2008a).

Both of these documents make clear the necessity for anti-oppressive, non-discriminatory practice as a core principle for all registered practitioners to ensure that they do not bring their profession into disrepute. The regulatory bodies state that practitioners should 'be open and honest, act with integrity and uphold the reputation of your profession' (Nursing and Midwifery Council 2008a:1) and 'Behave with integrity and honesty. Make sure your behaviour does not damage your profession's reputation' (Health Professions Council 2008a:1).

Reflective point

- As a leader and role model, do unprofessional and occasionally distasteful comments or gossip about colleague's gender, ethnicity, sexual orientation, religion or disability contravene your professional Code of Conduct?

Clear, unequivocal and specific legislation exists in order to prevent discrimination on the grounds of race, gender, sexual orientation, age, religious beliefs or disability, for example the Disability

Discrimination Act 2005, Age Discrimination Act 2006, Equality Act 2006, Gender Equality Act 2007, and Gender Recognition Act 2004, the last giving transsexual individuals the legal right to recognition of their acquired gender (all accessible at directgov.com). There is no shortage of information on the provision of these Acts, which are enshrined in law and should be respected and enforced.

Another instrument to combat oppressive behaviour is the ability of a manager. The skills required include knowing the job, being an excellent communicator, being a good role model, being able to set clear goals and being able to set outcomes for the team (Fincham & Rhodes 1999). A manager should be in touch with their team and be accessible to them. Bennis (1997:53) suggests that 'too much distance makes leadership like pornography . . . just a mechanical act'. A manager must know their team and know what is happening in their department. The most sought-after qualities that perioperative practitioners look for in a leader are fairness, integrity, professionalism, trustworthiness, approachability, ability to empower staff, honesty, good communication skills, clinical competence and good interpersonal skills (Dunn 2003).

> Reflective point
> • How many of those qualities would your team say you possess?

The Health Professions Council (2007a) has provided a very comprehensive guide to a disabled person's rights and needs in becoming a health professional. Each organization will also have its response to the Disability Discrimination Act 2005. This will reiterate the rights of disabled members of a team, including a section on making 'reasonable adjustments' in the working environment to empower a disabled person. The human resource department of the employer will refer a manager to the appropriate person within the administration to help in carrying out a risk assessment to ensure the rights of a disabled person while meeting the duty to protect the public.

The Nursing and Midwifery Council (2008a, 2008b) is also unequivocal in its support for equality on the grounds of race, gender, religion, sexual orientation and disability.

When there are specific problems arising from cultural differences, it is the manager's duty to deal with these problems and find solutions, particularly if these have an adverse impact on patient care.

Some common cultural conflicts

This discussion above is far from exhaustive but the following section highlights some of the topics that frequently arise in discussions on diversity in the perioperative environment.

Conflicts can arise when working with internationally recruited staff with poor command of English. The *Standards of Proficiency* of the Health Professions Council 2008b:8) states that aspirant registrants must 'be able to communicate at level 7 of the English language Testing System with no element below level 6.5'. The Code of Conduct (Nursing and Midwifery Council 2008a) and the *Standards of Conduct, Performance and Ethics* (Health Professions Council 2008a) state clearly that effective communication is essential for safe patient care.

If a problem of this type arises for a manager, the answer may lie in referral to 'English as a second language' classes, which are very often to been found free of charge in a local further education college. Cultural differences in the speed of physical movement expected in theatre need to be explained to practitioners from outside the prevailing culture. It is vital to explain that an apparently 'laid back' approach to responding to urgent perioperative situations can be misconstrued as being lazy.

People in Western cultures are thought to be more aggressive in their activity than Asians. It is common to disagree strongly with someone on single issues and yet remain friends. Westerners often place a great deal of weight on individual rights and achievements. By contrast, Asians tend to be more passive and defensive and they strive for social harmony;

consequently, they will try to avoid a public show of disagreement (Humayun Ansari & Jackson 1996).

There are some Asian cultures in which it would not be considered appropriate to offer even the least challenge to a doctor; in contrast, the culture and regulatory bodies in the UK dictate that nurses and operative department practitioners are the patients' advocate. Therefore, it is expected that such staff will speak up on any matter that concerns patients' physical and psychological wellbeing.

The Nursing and Midwifery Council (2008b) advises the use of supervised practice for nurses from outside the UK to ensure that they meet the standards of practice demanded for registration.

The Department of Health (2007) in its publication *The Positively Diverse Process* provides extensive details on maximizing the benefits of meeting the health needs of communities through the recruitment, development and retention of a workforce that reflects the diversity of the population. The policy initiative seeks also to ensure that the NHS is a fair employer offering 'equality of opportunity and outcomes in the workplace'.

Reflective points

- How would you cope with working in a foreign country where the language, social mores, food and working practices were unfamiliar?
- What would be your coping mechanisms if you were there alone and homesick?

The use of mentors in such problem situations is invaluable. 'Mentors are role models. Showing a new nurse a specific task is not the same as explaining why the task is performed and modelling the behaviour' Fawcett (2002:950). Clutterbuck (2004:3) enlarges on the role of mentors: 'Mentors provide a spectrum of learning and supporting behaviours, from challenging and being a critical friend to being a role model, from helping build networks and developing personal resourcefulness to simply being there to listen, from helping people work out what they want to achieve, and why, to planning how they will bring change about'.

If problems exist with the ability of any of the practitioners being managed, the same policies and procedures should apply, irrespective of differences in race, religion, gender, disability and sexual orientation (Thompson 1997).

1. Establish the facts concerning any alleged wrong doing, incorrect practice or misconduct.
2. Do this professionally and confidentially.
3. Follow the disciplinary procedures laid down by the organization.
4. Inform the line manager and take advice.
5. Seek guidance and advice from the human resource department, especially if this is a situation that has not been encountered previously.
6. Inform the individual who is subject of investigation what the issues are, what their rights are and refresh them on the details of the disciplinary procedures being used.
7. Avoid listening to gossip or encouraging it.
8. Collect facts from eye witnesses not from hearsay and opinions (both of which can be offered in generous amounts).
9. Approach the investigation into the alleged incident with an open mind.
10. Remember that in cases of gross misconduct it is usual to suspend the employee from the workplace while the enquiry is ongoing. This is to protect the interest of the employee and in some cases to protect the public.

Depending on the findings of the investigation, the manager, on behalf of the organization, has the following options.

1. Make the person who does not meet the required standards of performance in their role subject to the organization's 'capability' policy. This allows the individual to continue to work under close supervision. It sets explicit aims, objectives and time frames to help him or her to bring their work up to the required standard.
2. Refer to the appropriate professional regulatory body. If the person in question is a registered practitioner, there is a very clear pathway to follow in such a referral.
3. Refer the alleged misconduct to either a conduct and competence committee or a health

committee. The outcome may be a decision requiring suspension for a set period of time, referral for medical advice and possibly care, a time of retraining on areas of practice or removal from the register (Nursing and Midwifery Council 2008b; Health Professions Council 2007b). The simplest way for a manager to find out the particular cultural needs of the diverse members of their team is to ask them. It is incumbent on a manager to create a healthy working environment that fosters an atmosphere in which the talents of all the team are optimized to deliver the highest standards of care to the patients in the team's care.

Making a strength of diversity is compared by Herriot & Pemberton (1995:8–9) to culinary endeavours. The 'vindaloo' model of diversity assimilates everything into the dish, with a consequence that everything tastes the same. The 'nouvelle cuisine' approach treats diversity as a very delicate but apparently useless decoration on the side of the plate. The 'traditional English Sunday lunch' model amounts to all of the ingredients being of equal value in the success of the meal. Valuing diversity ensures that organizations have a competitive edge, a constant input of fresh ideas and new perspectives and a safe working environment where the energy and action is focused outwardly on patient care not inwardly on destructive, damaging and petty oppressive behaviour.

When it comes to eliminating oppressive practices, the choice for a manager is a simple one: be part of the solution not part of the problem.

REFERENCES

Advisory Conciliation Arbitration Service (2008). *Workplace Training Impact Survey*. London: Advisory Conciliation Arbitration Service; http://www.employment-studies.co.uk/summary/summary.php?id=acas0808 (accessed 5 May 2009).

BBC News (2006) *Study Reveals Nurse Bully Problem*. http://news.bbc.co.uk/1/hi/scotland/521 (accessed 5 May 2009).

Bennis, W. (1997). *Managing People is Like Herding Cats*. London: Kogan Page.

Bolchover, D. & Brady, C. (2004). *The 90-Minute Manager*. London: Pearson Prentice Hall.

Brown, A. (1998). *Organisational Culture*, 2nd edn. London: Prentice Hall.

Clutterbuck, D. (2004). *Everyone Needs a Mentor*, 4th edn. London: Chartered Institute Of Personnel and Development.

Concise Oxford Dictionary (1992). Oxford: Oxford University Press, p. 282.

Department of Health (2007). *The Positively Diverse Process*. London: The Stationery Office.

Dunn, H. (2003). Horizontal violence amongst nurses. *AORN Journal*, **78**, 977–988.

Esmail, A. (2005). Slow boat to equality. *The Guardian*, 31 November; http://www.guardian.co.uk (accessed 6 July 2008).

Fawcett, D. (2002). Mentoring: what it is and how to make it work. *AORN Journal*, **75**, 950–954.

Fincham, R. & Rhodes, P. (1999). *Principles of Organisational Behaviour*, 3rd edn. New York: Oxford University Press.

Fortunato, N. (2000). *Berry & Kohn's Operating Room Technique*, 9th edn. New York: Mosby.

Giga, S., Hoel, H. & Lewis, D. (2008). *A Review of Black and Minority Ethnic (BME) Employee Experiences of Workplace Bullying*. London: Dignity at Work Partnership.

Griffin, M. (2004). Teaching cognitive rehearsal as a shield for lateral violence: an intervention for newly licensed nurses. *Journal of Continuing Education in Nursing*, **35**, 257–263.

Hadikin, R. & O' Driscoll, M. (2000). *The Bullying Culture*. Edinburgh: Elsevier.

Health and Safety Executive (2005). *HSE condemns bullying in the workplace*. London: Health and Safety Executive; http://www.healthandsafetyexecutive.org.uk (accessed 25 May 2008).

Health Professions Council (2007a). *A Disabled Person's Guide to Becoming a Health Professional*. London: Health Professions Council.

Health Professions Council (2007b). *The Fitness to Practice Process*. London: Health Professions Council.

Health Professions Council (2008a). *Standards of Conduct, Performance and Ethics*. London: Health Professions Council.

Health Professions Council (2008b). *Standards of Proficiency*. Operating Department Practitioners. London: Health Professions Council.

Herriot, P. & Pemberton, C. (1995). *Competitive Advantage Through Diversity*. London: Sage.

Hoel, H., Sparks, K. & Cooper, C. L. (2001). *The Cost of Violence/Stress at Work. The Benefits of a Violence/Stress Free Working Environment.* Geneva: International Labour Organisation.

Humayun Ansari K. & Jackson J. (1996). *Managing Cultural Diversity at Work.* London: Kogan Page.

Kelly, J. (2006). An overview of conflict. *Dimensions of Critical Care Nursing*, **25**, 22–28.

McPherson W. (1999). *The Stephen Lawrence Inquiry* [McPherson Report]. London: The Stationery Office.

Morris, P. W. G. (2001). Updating the project management bodies of knowledge. *Project Management Journal*, **32**, 21–30.

Nursing and Midwifery Council (2008a). *The Code. Standards of Conduct, Performance and Ethics for Nurses and Midwives.* London: Nursing and Midwifery Council.

Nursing and Midwifery Council (2008b). *Standards to Support Learning and Assessment in Practice.* London: Nursing and Midwifery Council.

Patterson, P. (2007). Lateral violence. Why it's serious and what OR managers can do about it. *OR Manager*, **23**, 12.

Quine, L. (1999). Workplace bullying in NHS community trusts: staff questionnaire. *British Medical Journal*, **318**, 228–232.

Stanley, K. M., Dulaney, P. & Martin, M. M. (2007). Nurses 'eating our young' – it has a name: lateral violence. *South Carolina Nurse*, **14,** 17–18.

Stevens, S. (2002). Nursing workforce retention. challenging a workplace culture. *Health Affairs*, **21**, 189–193.

Taylor, K. (2004). Fear and loathing in the workplace. *The Guardian*, 8 July; http://www.guardian.co.uk (accessed 30 March 2008).

Templar, R. (2005). *The Rules of Management.* London: Pearson Prentice Hall.

The Phrase Finder (2008). http://www.phrases.org.uk/ (accessed 20 April 2009).

Thompson, R. (1997). *Managing People*, 2nd edn. London: Butterworth Heinmann.

USEFUL WEBSITES COVERING BULLYING AT WORK

Andrea Adams Trust 01273704900. www.andreadamstrust.org.

Commission for Racial Equality www.cre.gov.uk.

Disability Rights Commission www.drc.org.

Samaritans www.samaritans.org.

8

Leadership in perioperative settings: a practical guide

Ian Cumming

Key Learning Points

- Appreciate what good leadership is, and what it is not
- Understand the nature of leadership and whether it is a quality that can be taught or learned
- Appreciate the qualities of established leaders
- Identify ways of improving leadership in perioperative settings

People often misunderstand and misuse the terms leadership and management. It is possible to be a good leader without being a manager, or even without having the word management in a job description. Equally, it is possible for a person to be a successful manager without the team perceiving that person to be a leader. The question is what exactly is the difference between leadership and management. There are many ways to distinguish between management and leadership and the following is my preferred definition.

Management is about tasks, systems and processes; leadership is about people. You lead a team and manage a bank account. Leadership is about identifying and delivering a vision.

Leadership is, therefore, about people and about developing and communicating a vision; it is also about creating an environment in which everyone works towards a common goal or objective. To be successful, a leader does not require formal academic learning or training in management techniques (although many may choose to aim for these). The most important point to remember is that a leader cannot be a leader without followers.

Whether good leaders are born or created is a debate that runs and runs. My view is that it is both. I agree with John Adair's (1979) view that nobody can teach leadership: it is something that leaders learn principally from experience and practice, which is illuminated by principles and ideas.

This chapter explores seven key principles or skills that leaders need to become a successful leader in healthcare. However, leadership cannot be taught with a book; leaders will also require experience, practice and feedback on their performance from others.

Leading a team

John Adair (1979), in his Action Centred Leadership Model, describes the successful team leader as spending leadership time on three distinct parts. The first is focused on delivering the task. The second is focused on the interrelationships between team members to make sure that everybody is working together to deliver the maximum that the team can. Finally, the third part is focused on each team member's own needs or desires. When reflecting on how much time a team leader spends on each of these three areas, most people find that most of their time is devoted to delivering the 'task'.

Core Topics in Operating Department Practice: Leadership and Management, ed. Brian Smith, Paul Rawling, Paul Wicker and Chris Jones. Published by Cambridge University Press. © Cambridge University Press 2010.

Within busy working lives, and especially within front-line healthcare, it is far too easy for leaders to focus on achieving the task – be that finishing an operating list on time, meeting targets or ensuring the best possible clinical outcome – at the expense of other aspects of leading a team. While focusing on the task is important, the leader should also consider the needs of individuals within a team and the dynamics within the team. Otherwise, at best there will be an unhappy working environment; at worst not achieving the task and, therefore, patient care will suffer.

Adair (1979) argues that successful leaders will split their time equally. They should spend a third of available time as leader on delivering the task. A second third of the time should be spent on the dynamics between individuals within the team and making sure the team as a whole is working to its maximum potential. The leader should spend the final third of the time talking to, developing and understanding the individuals within the team.

> **Reflective point**
>
> - Do you spend equal amounts of your time on the task, the team and the individuals within that team? Forget the latter two at your peril.

Leadership styles

There are many examples of successful leaders who yet have differed in leadership style. Mahatma Ghandi, Winston Churchill and Nelson Mandela, for example, are all seen as successful leaders, but with different styles and approaches to leadership. In the same way, individual leaders within the healthcare environment all have their own preferred style. Despite having a preferred style, good leaders need to be able to develop different styles for different occasions.

Daniel Goleman (2000) has written extensively on emotional intelligence and leadership styles,

Table 8.1 Leadership styles

Leadership style	Description
Affiliative	Creates harmony and builds emotional bonds
Authoritative	Mobilizes people towards a vision
Coaching	Develops people for the future
Democratic	Consensus through participation of all
Pace-setting	Sets and expects high standards of performance (use with caution, see text)
Coercive	Demands immediate compliance (use with caution, see text)

Source: Goleman (2000).

arguing that successful leaders should be able to move seamlessly between six leadership styles, as the situation dictates (Table 8.1).

For example, different clinical situations require different leadership styles. During an emergency, for example a cardiac arrest, a *democratic* leadership style from the person leading the resuscitation may be disastrous for the patient. In this clinical situation, because of the critical time factor, an *authoritative* leadership style is essential: issuing tasks and instructions to individuals. This style might even have to move to *coercive* if, for example, an individual was not doing as requested. Moving on in time, and assuming that the resuscitation had been successful, the leadership style would need to change. Some people involved in the resuscitation might be upset or frightened; others may want to discuss why the leader acted in a particular fashion. A good leader would at this stage change leadership style, possibly into a *coaching* style to explore learning from the event. Did it go as well as it could? Did everyone play their part and understand what was going on? An *affiliative* style might also be needed to bring the team together, especially if the resuscitation had been unsuccessful.

In this clinical example, the leader moved through several different leadership styles

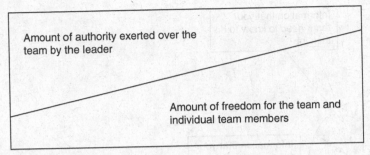

Figure 8.1 The Tannenbaum and Schmidt (1973) continuum.

responding to the circumstance that they faced. The same principles apply in non-clinical leadership situations. Working on a day-to-day basis, most leaders have a preferred or 'natural' leadership style. There is nothing wrong with this. Good leaders should be aware, however, that their preferred style will not work in all situations. Successful leaders must develop different styles. It is usually hard for people to develop the coercive, dictatorial style if that is not the way they naturally behave; however, it can be done. Also, it is hard for people who are naturally coercive to suddenly become inclusive and use a democratic style. Good leaders would think about their natural leadership style and, when fitting, may try using one or more of the other styles.

Coercive and pace-setting leadership styles must be used with caution. The coercive style is commonly used in the military where absolute compliance with orders is required. While this style can be suitable in civilian life, these occasions are rare. The coercive leadership style is often linked closely with arrogance as a leadership trait (see below). This combination does not allow for challenge or comment on the leader's perspective and can, therefore, be dangerous as team members may not speak up to prevent errors being made.

Pace setting also needs to be used with caution because demotivation, stress and burnout can occur if an individual sets such high personal standards and such a high level of productivity that others are unable to keep up.

Delegation and development

It would be inappropriate to leave a discussion about leadership styles without considering the areas of delegation and development of team members. Learning how and what to delegate is a key developmental area for many leaders. Delegation is not about passing mundane or unpleasant tasks on to others simply because the leader does not want to do them. Successful leaders never delegate anything that they are unwilling to do themselves. Delegation should be seen as a fair way of dividing tasks, but also as a way of developing individual members of the team and, therefore, the team as a whole. Once the leader has delegated the task, the right balance also needs to be struck between letting people feel abandoned and out of their depth and letting them feel that the leader is sitting watching their every move. Remember, people are all individuals and some people will want more support than others; it is up to the leader to get to know the individual members of the team.

The Tannenbaum & Schmidt (1973) continuum is a model that shows the relationship between the amounts of freedom that a team has and the authority exerted over that team by its leader. The continuum is probably best pictured using a diagram (Fig. 8.1). As you can see, the less authority that the leader displays over the team, the more freedom the team members have to act. Over time, successful leaders will ensure that their teams move along the continuum to the right. High-performing

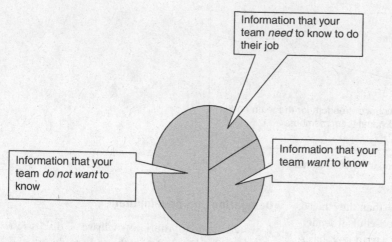

Figure 8.2 Distribution of knowledge in a team.

teams are on the right-hand end of the continuum; they will also have developed one or two potential successors to the team leader.

> **Reflective points**
>
> - Can you define your preferred leadership style (ask others to help)?
> - Are there other styles that could be used in suitable circumstances?
> - How, what and why do you delegate?

Communication

Communication is often highlighted within many medium and large organizations as an area in which performance could be much improved. If there is poor communication within a team, then 50% of the fault for this lies with the team leader – the other 50% is balanced among the team members. Good communication is always the result of a two-way process.

Communicating with the team is not simply about talking to them. The old adage 'you have two eyes, two ears, and one mouth and they should be used in that proportion' is true when it comes to how leaders communicate with their teams. A good leader must ensure that systems are in place for briefing team members, but team members also have a responsibility to ask questions. Leaders, as well as having a responsibility for communicating with their teams, also have a responsibility for ensuring good communication between the team and the rest of the organization. Good leaders never say to their team 'I don't know what's going on; no one tells me anything'; they find out what they need to know.

Deciding how and what to communicate to the team can be a challenge for any leader. Individual team members often have different views on how much they want to know, for example about what is happening elsewhere in the organization.

Consider the pie chart in Fig. 8.2. The complete pie represents all the information available to the team. Only some of this is information that an individual *needs* to know to do their job. In almost all circumstances, this information is communicated. If it were not, the job simply would not get done. The second section of the pie represents the information that an individual *wants* to know, for example about their job or their workplace. This is the area where many teams fail with communication. Not communicating what people want to know leads to a knowledge gap. People may fill knowledge gaps with rumour and speculation. Rumour and speculation will eventually always have an adverse impact on morale and motivation within the team. Leaders need to find out what their team members want to know and then communicate it to them. Leaders should also encourage their teams to ask them questions. If leaders do not know the answer, then it is incumbent on them to find out and go back with the answer. The final section of the pie, described as 'irrelevant information', is worthy of some consideration too. In an attempt to be a good communicator, some leaders pass on to their team everything that they possibly can whether it is of any relevance or interest to team members or not. Regularly communicating information that the team members have no wish to know can be just as bad as failing to communicate, as people will simply stop listening. Use of e-mail communications, and 'cc' and 'reply to all', are often to blame for this.

A fundamental part of communicating with team members is giving and receiving feedback. Feedback is a powerful tool in improving the performance of the team leader and the team members, plus that of the team overall. While I am a great supporter of formal feedback mechanisms, I want to concentrate here on giving and receiving informal feedback – perhaps at the end of a day or over a cup of coffee. If feedback is never given, how does the team know if it is doing a good, a bad or an indifferent job?

Looking at positive feedback first, consider how often a leader says thank you to their team (while meaning it). Highly-performing teams receive regular affirmation from their leader that they are doing a good job. This boosts team morale and individual motivation, leading to a happier team and improved performance.

Conversely, badly given feedback about areas in which an individual could improve is hugely demoralizing and causes defensive behaviour rather than any improvement. There are a few good principles for giving and receiving feedback.

Leaders must consider carefully what they are going to say before saying it. For example, saying 'Well you made a mess of that didn't you!' is not feedback, it is criticism. It may be useful for leaders to consider how they would like to receive feedback if they were a team member in that situation. A better approach would be – at a suitable time and place – to explain to the individual the particular behaviour trait that was displayed, illustrating with a specific occasion when they demonstrated this trait, and then explain why behaving differently might produce a better/different outcome.

When receiving feedback, think of it as a present. Whenever people are given a present – whether it is wanted or not – they always respond with a 'thank you'. The same should be done when receiving feedback. It is difficult not to become defensive; however, feedback is only one person's perception of that behaviour and it may be inaccurate. As with a present (such as a vase), there are three choices about what to do with feedback: ignore it (throw it away), store it away for future reference or ask others for advice (put it in a cupboard) or decide to act on it there and then (put it on display). Feedback should not be ignored. An old Arabic proverb can be loosely translated as 'if one person tells you that you are a camel, laugh; if two people tell you that you are a camel think about it, and if three people tell you that you are camel, buy a saddle!'.

Leaders who find that they are getting no feedback about their performance should ask themselves why. Is the culture of the team such that feedback is frowned upon? Is the team frightened of the leader? Will your team only tell the leader what he or she wants to hear? In this situation, leaders should try asking for feedback – they might be surprised at what comes back. Alternatively, leaders can use a properly facilitated feedback instrument (ideally 360 degree feedback) to seek the views of others on their performance and other's perceptions of the team's performance.

Reflective points

- How do you communicate with your team?
- How much is 'talking at' as opposed to 'listening to'?
- Find out what your team want to know and how they want to be communicated with. Encourage giving and receiving feedback.

Strategic planning (creating a vision)

How do you know when you have arrived if you don't know where you are going? Every successful team and every good leader have a vision for what they are trying to achieve. The team must consider the following six basic steps:

1. Decide where they want to be and what they want to achieve
2. Consider how they are going to get there
3. Make a plan
4. Consider what might go wrong to stop them achieving their objectives
5. Set intermediate objectives (milestones) to measure progress
6. Measure against those objectives until the outcome is reached.

The key to successful strategic thinking is that it cannot be carried out alone. This is not the time for a coercive leadership style. The leader's job is to merge the top-down thinking from outside the team with the bottom-up thinking coming from the team itself. The successful leader has a key role to play in identifying the vision, but then an even more important role in communicating it and ensuring that the team delivers it.

Reflective points

- Strategy is not something that is only the province of directors. How can you set a good strategy?
- Do you discuss with your team what you want to achieve and how you are going to achieve it?
- Do you set milestones to measure progress?

Managing change

Change is a fact of life in healthcare. Even if the political and policy drivers for change in healthcare were to subside, which is unlikely, demographic changes, technological advances and changes in the epidemiology of disease are all going to have an enormous impact on how healthcare is delivered and how healthcare workers work over the next few years. Those working in healthcare typically feel that change is continually imposed on them against their wishes. This can be an important factor in team performance. When faced with significant enforced change, the emotional response in an individual or team is similar to that seen following a sudden bereavement – first sadness, then anger, then resentment and then finally acceptance (or SARA for short).

How quickly individuals or teams move through these phases of emotional response depends on the significance of the change but also on the ability of the leader to galvanize the team and to move on.

If change comes about because of 'our idea', the person or team who had the idea likes it, embraces it and implements it. If the whole team is 'on board' with the change and it is handled properly, this sort of change is a great boost to morale and motivation. This is clearly a much more positive position to be in than that of enforced change.

There are several approaches that a good leader can use to deal with enforced change. For example, the leader can try to 'change the change' into a change that the team can control. This way, the team has ownership and the change feels less imposed. To be able to deliver this requires a leader who is 'horizon scanning' outside the team to identify potential changes or new policies, for example in working practices. Once identified, the idea or policy should be discussed within the team and the team should agree how to implement it, rather than wait for an imposed solution.

Two final thoughts about managing change. The first is that the leader should be aware of 'cosmetic change'. This is where the team lets the leader believe that a change has been introduced when in reality things are carrying on just as before. This is surprisingly common, especially for enforced changes to working practices. The leader should make sure that he or she is involved enough to know whether or not change is really being implemented. The second thought is to not be afraid of 'noise'. 'Noise' includes, for example, complaints, grumbles, emails, letters or telephone calls. For major change, even with full involvement and acceptance from the team, there will be noise. Usually the quantity of noise is directly proportional to the significance of the change being introduced. No noise may well mean that no change is actually happening, or that the change is cosmetic. (See Ch. 19 for further discussion on change management.)

> **Reflective points**
>
> - Try to spot change – or the need for change – before change is imposed.
> - How would you and your team prefer to implement any change? Understanding this can alter an enforced change into team-led change.

Personal traits

There is an extensive amount of literature on the personal characteristics displayed by good leaders (Goleman 2000, Bennis & Goldsmith 2003). Table 8.2 summarizes seven key traits that need to be demonstrated in leaders and the effects of not doing so.

The first traits good leaders show is enthusiasm. Good leaders need to be enthusiastic about both the organization that they work for and what they and their team are trying to deliver. Maintaining a motivated team is impossible if the leader is constantly complaining about the NHS for example, or indeed other departments in the same organization.

A good leader also needs to be interested and committed to improving their team's performance, not just delivering the status quo. A high-performing team will not remain a high-performing team for long unless the team strives for continual improvement.

Good leaders also need to display a degree of toughness because a good leader cannot always be popular. Rather than striving to be popular, good leaders should aim to be respected for making fair decisions that are in the best interests of the team and the team's overall objectives. Being seen as fair does not mean, however, that the leader always has

Table 8.2 Traits of good leaders

Trait	If trait not displayed (a bad leader)
Enthusiasm	Will show a lack of interest in team and the task
Commitment	Will give up when the going gets tough
Toughness: seeks respect rather than popularity	Will avoid difficult decisions to remain popular; tolerates poor performance
Fairness	Will treat team members unfairly; have favourites
Humility	Will be arrogant, always knowing best; will be a 'control freak'
Confidence	Will be risk averse; may be too cautious
Integrity/trust	Will be untrustworthy

to treat everyone within the team in the same way. No two people are the same and, therefore, no two people will necessarily be treated in the same way.

The next trait is harder to describe. It is impossible to be a good leader if the leader is arrogant. The opposite of arrogance is humility (defined by the *Oxford English Dictionary* as 'taking a humble view of one's own importance'). Showing humility will undoubtedly make for a better leader. Good leaders allow their team to take the credit for successes but are quick to put themselves forward at times of failure. Catherine the Great (1729–1796) summed this up in two short sentences: 'I praise loudly. I blame softly'.

Leaders need to be confident, but they must beware of becoming overconfident as overconfidence leads to arrogance. Finally, leaders need to be seen by others as a person with integrity and a person who can be trusted.

> **Reflective points**
>
> - What are your traits?
> - Do you complain to your team about your employer?
> - Do you think you are perceived as arrogant?
> - Do you always strive to be popular? If so, think about the impact that behaving differently might produce, and try it.

Conclusions

'Morale is at an all-time low!' Many people will have heard this within the perioperative environment in recent years. Undoubtedly, this will result partly from enforced change, poor communication, lack of direction and too much focus on delivering the task, or in other words, as explored above, poor leadership. There is more to it than just blaming the leader though. A successful team is not just about having a good leader; it is also about having motivated and enthusiastic team members.

There are two sorts of people in society: those who have a 'can do' attitude and those who have a 'can't do' attitude. Not surprisingly, both sets of people get exactly what they believe. There are many instances where suggestions for working differently have been met by individuals committing significant amounts of time and effort into looking at all the reasons why it will not work or cannot be done. If just some of this time was spent on embracing the idea and looking at how it could be done and how it could be made to work, think what impact that would have on a team's morale and motivation. While on the subject of morale, the easiest way of driving down morale is by talking about how bad morale is. Team leaders should try to focus on the positive aspects of the job and be optimistic about the future. Who knows it may become contagious!

Reflective points

- Develop a can do attitude both within and without your team.
- Be optimistic about the future.

The **Key Learning Points** for developing leadership skills can be summarized as follows:

- spend equal amounts of time on the task, the team and the individuals within that team
- define your preferred leadership style but consider other styles in appropriate circumstances
- think about how, what and why you delegate
- consider how you communicate with your team, how well you listen as well as speak
- find out how much your team wants to know and how they want to be communicated with
- encourage giving and receiving feedback
- set strategy by discussing with your team what you want to achieve and how you are going to achieve it, setting milestones to measure progress
- look out for change or the need for change so you are aware of this before it is imposed; help the team to think about how change will be implemented and so make enforced changes into team-led changes
- consider your own traits and the impacts they might have on the team and whether you need to change
- develop a 'can do' attitude both within and without your team and foster an optimistic attitude.

Note

Much of the content of this chapter has derived from Cumming, I. (2008) *The Little Black Book of Leadership Hints and Tips for Healthcare Staff*. Littleborough: Perfect Circle. © NHS North Lancashire/Ian Cumming. Please refer to this for further reading.

REFERENCES

Adair, J. (1979). *Action Centred Leadership*. London: Gower.

Bennis, W. & Goldsmith, J. (2003). *Learning to Lead: A Workbook on Becoming a Leader*. New York: Perseus Books.

Goleman, D. (2000). *Leadership that Gets Results*. Boston, MA: Harvard Business Review.

Tannenbaum, R. & Schmidt, W. H. (1973). *How to Choose a Leadership Pattern*. Boston, MA: Harvard Business Review.

9

Management and leadership of advanced practice

Judith Roberts

Key Learning Points

- Understand the different drivers for the development of advanced roles
- Examine the common characteristics of an advanced role
- Define advanced practice and examination of the common characteristics of advanced roles
- Understand the issues involved in management of advanced practitioners and leadership of a team to advance the quality of service

Introduction

One of the defining characteristics of living in the twenty-first century is adapting to the changes that have been prompted by evolving technological, political, economic and social developments.

Healthcare practice has not been immune to these influences (World Health Organization 2002, 2006). Comparing current healthcare practice with that of the 1970s reveals a whole career's worth of development and adaptation to these differing patterns of disease and healthcare provision. An operating department manager and leader must recognize this fact (Kay 2005) and not only deal with its impact but, more importantly, also proactively anticipate possible changes or shifts of emphasis so that manager and team are able to adapt and meet the opportunities and challenges they may pose (Dubois *et al.* 2006).

The PEST analysis

The PEST analysis (**p**olitical, **e**conomic, **s**ocial and **t**echnological factors; QuickMBA 2008) is one way of considering the impact of various factors on the role of the advanced practitioner.

There has been no single revolutionary force promoting the development of the non-medically qualified advanced practitioner. The origins of the advanced practitioner have been much more evolutionary, organic and complex, as healthcare systems worldwide have risen to the combined challenges presented by these external forces.

Advances in medicine and diagnostics, for example new drugs, treatments and techniques, are part of the reason why people are living longer in general, although it is recognized that this increased lifespan is often accompanied by an increased morbidity, especially in the later years of life (National Statistics 2006).

The days when a patient commonly had only one named condition and only one potential complication are now in the past. Currently, there are now more patients with more complex conditions having more complex treatments than ever before (Department of Health 2005). Within a healthcare service, including the operating department, this translates to an increased volume of referrals for treatments and increased clinical acuity of the patient group, which increases clinical risk; this has a dramatic effect on national healthcare expenditure.

Core Topics in Operating Department Practice: Leadership and Management, ed. Brian Smith, Paul Rawling, Paul Wicker and Chris Jones. Published by Cambridge University Press. © Cambridge University Press 2010.

As treatment options advance, the skills needed to manage the patient population clinically are also more advanced. It is thought that this situation has been one of the catalysts for the development of new advanced practitioner roles (Cameron 2000).

Socially, patient expectations and lifestyles have also created a demand, partially fuelled and endorsed by government policy (Department of Health 2006a). The public now commonly expects a shorter waiting time for hospital appointments, treatments that require less-invasive procedures and an accompanied shorter stay in hospital (Scholes 2006).

In summary there have been broadly two interconnected reasons why there is an increased demand for healthcare: increased service demands and policy demands.

Increased service demands

Increased service demands arise from demographic, awareness and technological factors. Demographically, there is a larger volume of patients requiring treatments. People are living longer but with increased healthcare needs. This creates additional clinical demand, especially as people are generally better informed about treatment options and are more skilled at requesting them. Research and clinical innovations (surgical, technological and pharmacological) combined with service developments have increased the treatment options that are now recommended by relevant national service frameworks, local care pathways and governance protocols.

Policy demands

The economic impact of the UK's changed demographics is not to be underestimated (Wanless 2004) as the Department of Health (2008) states that 'people with limiting long term conditions are the most intensive users of the most expensive services'. It is a stark and blunt fact that ill health is far more costly to the NHS purse than early mortality. This is why the health promotion agenda

proposed in the Wanless Report is so vital yet, as it acknowledges, costly. This is because the health promotion effort has to be funded while concurrently funding the healthcare consequences of current unhealthy lifestyles.

These changes have all occurred within a modernizing health service dominated (quite rightly) by a governance with a performance management agenda (Department of Health 2000, 2004a, 2004b). In such a situation, when there are so many financial demands on the nation's health service, there is little room for waste. Therefore, organizations are expected to be both effective and efficient, thus providing the same outcomes for less expenditure or improved outcomes for the same cost, or, best of all, improved outcomes for reduced expenditure. Some of these expectations have been set as operational targets; relevant to the surgical and perioperative sector is the *18 Week Patient Pathway* work streams (Department of Health 2006b).

Impact of reduction in working hours of doctors

Importantly, this increased demand for healthcare services, heightened clinical expertise and service improvement has emerged *at the same time* as the reduction in working hours for junior doctors to meet the European Working Time Directive. This reduction has been further exacerbated by the changes to junior medical training programmes resulting from *Modernising Medical Careers* (Department of Health 2004c). Additionally other changes to GP contracts and out-of-hours services have all hampered the day-to-day deployment of sufficient numbers of suitably qualified clinical practitioners. A summary of these issues is given in Fig. 9.1.

The UK Government, no doubt influenced by the development of advanced practitioners in the USA, recognized that other professional groups could start to work differently and thus act as substitutes for the 'missing' doctors. Consequently, a whole raft of policy initiatives gained momentum although, as summarized by Mantzoukas & Watkinson (2006),

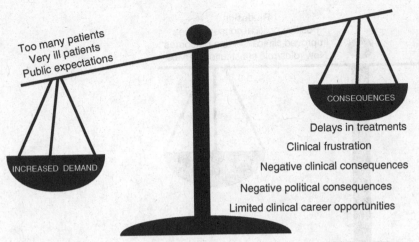

Too many patients
Very ill patients
Public expectations

INCREASED DEMAND

CONSEQUENCES

Delays in treatments

Clinical frustration

Negative clinical consequences

Negative political consequences

Limited clinical career opportunities

Figure 9.1 Consequences of not managing increased healthcare demands.

confusion still exists around the different interpretation of titles and roles.

At the time of writing, proposed changes to nurse education and post-registration career pathways are open for consultation. One of the purposes of these reviews is to address the current and future education and registration requirements of practitioners, with the aim of preparing registrants for a demanding clinical career in which clinical complexity, governance and application of technology will be key features.

Since the late 1990s and early part of the twenty-first century, non-medically qualified healthcare practitioners have demonstrated their ability, capacity and willingness to take on further training and development to substitute for doctors, within both community and acute settings (Laurant *et al.* 2004, Davies 2006, Rushforth *et al.* 2006, Cox & Hall 2007). In the process, they have also initiated new services, improved outdated systems and developed new skills (Fig. 9.2).

As the Department of Health (2006c) recognizes, meeting the requirements of the European Working Time Directive has been a serendipitous opportunity to modernize the service, ultimately being a real catalyst for change. Significantly, however, it must be remembered that these developments would not have happened if practitioners themselves had not been prepared to take on these new roles.

It is safe to say (in 2008) that, in this more clinically governed NHS, it is very likely that if these new practitioners had demonstrated significantly poorer outcomes this chapter would not have been written, for anecdotal evidence, critical incidents, professional bodies and even coroner reports would have prompted a swift end of the development, far in advance of any research findings. Nonetheless, it is worth heeding Paterson's (1998) warning that legal and ethical aspects of practice will require more reflection as practice becomes more complex and demanding. This is echoed by Cooke's (2006) concerns that as new roles are developed proper research strategies should be used to evaluate their impact thoroughly, while also undertaking rigorous audit and evaluation to ensure that clinical safety and quality healthcare are still being maintained and that practitioners perform to an 'adequate standard'.

Back in 2001, Bishop & Scott (2001:12) posed this interesting question: 'how can the NHS provide individualised patient care that is user centred and meets the demands of a knowledgeable and litigious society in an economy showing little sign of expansion?' Analysis of this quote and a full examination of all of the solutions is beyond the scope of this chapter but, as outlined above, the partial answer to this question has been to use a performance management, clinical governance

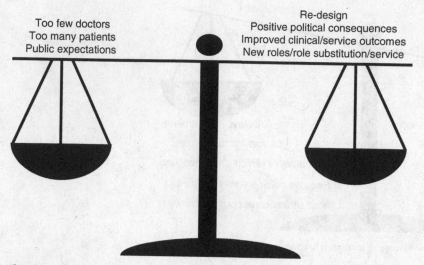

Figure 9.2 New roles: doctor substitution and service redesign.

approach to improve service provision, essentially through service redesign and service improvement combined often with staff developing and using new skills. Altogether, this is intended to improve the capacity and capability of staff and services as embodied in the Dimension G7: Capacity and Capability of *The NHS Knowledge and Skills Framework* (Department of Health 2004d).

This strategy is summarized below, although it must be recognized that this is a rather simplistic depiction of a complex situation.

The advanced practitioner strategy

Definitions

After a number of years of evolution and debate, the Nursing and Midwifery Council (2006) produced a definition of the advanced practitioner:

Advanced nurse practitioners are highly experienced, knowledgeable and educated members of the care team who are able to diagnose and treat your health care needs or refer you to an appropriate specialist if needed.

Currently, being a relatively new profession, there is little or no guidance about advanced practice

for operating department practitioners (ODPs). However, this will change as the profession becomes embedded and its horizons start to expand. In the meantime, it is likely that ODPs undertaking advanced roles will probably follow the same development route and have similar opportunities within the operating department as nurses.

Within the surgical and preoperative domains, advanced practitioners are often involved in the following roles or activities, doing some or all of the example activities:

patient group/ case management:	developing plans in collaboration with others, coordinating programmes of care, admitting/discharging patients, running clinics
clinical management:	undertaking history taking and clinical examinations, making diagnoses, screening patients, ordering investigations
performing surgical/investigative procedures:	endoscopy, working as surgical or anaesthetic assistants, working in surgical outreach teams
organizational activity:	leadership, educating staff, initiating research.

However, there are so many different definitions, national and international (International Council of Nurses 2003), and new roles for advanced health-care practitioners that trying to find a comprehensive definition is perhaps unnecessary and best left to the remit of human resources departments, the job description and the *Agenda for Change* job profile outline and NHS KSF outline (Department of Health 2004d).

Nonetheless, there is one consistent issue that remains within the domain of most advanced practitioners. Within the context of all healthcare staff working within policies, procedures and legislation (that are employer, national and professionally originated), it is the defining characteristic of an advanced practitioner that they make autonomous clinical decisions without deferment to any other professional. It is a further characteristic that these actions are only retrospectively monitored via clinical governance activities (e.g. case study review, audit activities, peer review and clinical supervision, user feedback, and critical event analysis).

This perspective is supported by MacDonald (2005), who found in her research (admittedly based within the community setting) that the ability to 'negotiate for autonomy' with GPs and other doctors was the significant feature of those working at a higher level of practice. 'Professional autonomy' also featured as an aspect of enhanced practice-based provision in the research findings of Mantzougas & Watkinson (2006).

Management and leadership issues

Advanced practice can be both a verb and a noun. An operating department manager may well be considering how to manage the advanced practitioners but may also be hoping to lead the team to support the advancement of the practice of both the manager and the team.

To avoid duplication with the other chapters in this book what will follow will be an exploration of issues and prompts to stimulate thoughts, with further reading and opportunities for further study.

Improving the quality of service

A manager may well be satisfied already by the perioperative service that is offered, but this opinion must be based on factual evidence and not just on an analysis of how hard the team is working.

However, teams often have to work harder to compensate for too few members. Occasionally, people need to work longer to cover for unexpected sickness and absence, and this is to be expected within any dynamic workplace. However if staffing shortages become entrenched then it is certainly demanding, if not too demanding, to provide a quality clinically safe service.

Rafferty *et al.* (2007) demonstrate a clear link between adequate staffing ratios and clinical safety outcomes, citing research that noted that those hospitals with poorer ratios of staff to patients had more than 25% higher mortality. Additionally, in those settings with poorer patient to staff ratios, it was reported that staff were twice as likely to have low morale and be dissatisfied with their jobs. This work specifically looked at ratios of nurses to patients but within the perioperative sector it could well also include ODPs. As the NHS Modernisation Agency (2005) states, 'A competent and committed workforce is a key requirement of a quality service'.

Therefore one of the main activities of an operating department manager may well be to ensure that there are adequate numbers of appropriately qualified people employed to meet the volume and complexity of the work. This will mean monitoring data that will demonstrate both the effectiveness (e.g. lack of critical incidents) and efficiency (e.g. volume of patients treated) of the department, since it has been demonstrated there is a causal link between the two (Dubois *et al.* 2006).

Not all staff development, however, needs to be formal or external to the unit (Price 2007), since there are many opportunities within the operating department to develop worthwhile in-house development programmes, for example through workshops (Nightingale 2007), or clinical supervision and mentoring (Scholes 2006).

How the manager and the team face up to the challenges of meeting service demands says a lot about the culture that operates both internally within the team and within the wider hospital management. Additionally, as McSherry (2004) indicates, both practice development and healthcare governance are also inextricably linked.

Initiating the role of advanced practitioner

Managing the advanced practitioner

There are many considerations to take into account if a manager decides to develop the role of advanced practitioner in a department. An important first step is to analyse and discuss with others the reasons why this role is needed. What is hoped to be the impact of the appointment? Are the expectations realistic in light of the number of people employed in the role and their power to influence and direct changes in practice. It will be crucial to consider the possible disadvantages if the new appointee will be a lone 'advanced' practitioner rather than part of a team, which ideally shares the workload and can offer personal and clinical support. Lone advanced practitioners will have few points of reference for their role, and may find themselves isolated in terms of practice and education. Professional and social isolation may result in higher stress levels.

The manager will also have to come to terms with the potential opportunities and challenges to their own job; the manager is likely to be developing the advanced skills of a manager not a practitioner. However, role bereavement may make the manager resent the new colleague, especially if he or she is taking over aspects of the manager's role that he or she previously enjoyed.

Practicalities in setting up an advanced practitioner role

The original bid for the advanced practitioner role must include a cost–benefit analysis with agreement on the problem, the solution and the informed expectations of the impact of the role. Ideally, current practice should be measured before the appointment or change so that the outcomes can be properly evaluated.

The job description must be accurate and precise, with further interpretation provided by the *Agenda for Change* job profile and NHS KSF outline.

Ideally there should be an assessment centre style of interview, including, if required, practical demonstrations of skill or at least use of clinical scenarios so that applicants can demonstrate their application of critical thinking, clinical knowledge and evidence-based practice.

Once an advanced practitioner is appointed, it will be necessary to continue to audit and monitor the practitioner's output as part of normal governance procedures and probably more frequently during their first year or so. Working autonomously in clinically challenging roles is not something that develops quickly; therefore, it must be recognized that moving from competent to expert, using Benner's (1984) model, will take time.

Conclusions

I am convinced that modernizing the NHS is not just about healthcare practitioners being able to undertake advanced clinical skills and tasks competently (as in the clinical specialist or practitioner roles), it also has to be about health practitioners, and consequently health professionals, thinking and behaving differently to achieve optimum healthcare outcomes for patients and their families. I believe that, as the world gets more complex and as patients, the public and politicians get more demanding, healthcare practitioners will need to be able to use information technology effectively. They need to be able to access and consider the plethora of information with discrimination and exercised judgement.

But knowledge and information technology are not all. We work in a human business: fallible humans working with fallible human beings.

Patients' needs should be at the centre of our efforts. Coping with life events and/or ill health can be frightening, tiring and, at times, an uncomfortable messy business.

I passionately believe that professional expertise is something that is visible by the absence of disharmony. The perfect team balances its priorities and values its individuals, and the result is that homeostasis is achieved. The dimensions of skilled practice look effortless, if not hidden, to the novice. But the patient knows how 'a real' practitioner makes them feel. As Reid (2001:22) states: 'it's the hidden bits that make it whole . . .'.

REFERENCES

Benner, P. (1984). *From Novice to Expert. Excellence and Power in Clinical Nursing Practice.* Menlo Park, CA: Addison-Wesley.

Bishop, V. & Scott, I. (2001). *Challenges in Clinical Practice.* Basingstoke: Palgrave.

Cameron, A. (2000). New role development in context. In Masterson, A. & Humphris, D. (eds.) *Developing New Clinical Roles: A Guide for Health Professionals,* pp. 7–24. Edinburgh: Churchill Livingstone.

Cooke, M. (2006). Emergency care practitioners: a new safe effective role? *Quality and Safety in Health Care,* **15**, 387–388.

Cox, C. & Hall, A. (2007). The advanced practice role in gastrointestinal nursing. *Gastrointestinal Nursing,* **5**, 26–31.

Davis, J. (2006). Setting up the role of emergency surgical nurse practitioner. *Journal of Perioperative Practice,* **16**, 144–147.

Department of Health (2000). *The NHS Plan: A Plan for Investment, a Plan for Reform.* London: The Stationery Office.

Department of Health (2004a). *Standards for Better Health.* London: The Stationery Office.

Department of Health (2004b). NHS *Improvement Plan: Putting People at the Heart of Public Services.* London: The Stationery Office.

Department of Health (2004c). *Modernising Medical Careers: The Next Steps.* London: The Stationery Office.

Department of Health (2004d). *The NHS Knowledge and Skills Framework (NHS KSF) and the Development Review Process.* London: The Stationery Office.

Department of Health (2005). *Supporting People with Long Term Conditions: An NHS and Social Care Model to Support Local Innovation and Integration.* London: The Stationery Office.

Department of Health (2006a). *Our Health, Our Care, Our Say: A New Direction for Community Services.* London: The Stationery Office.

Department of Health (2006b). *Tackling Hospital Waiting: The 18 Week Patient Pathway – An Implementation Framework.* London: The Stationery Office.

Department of Health (2006c). *European Working Time Directive.* London: The Stationery Office; http://www.dh.gov.uk/en/Policyandguidance/Humanresourcesand training/Modernisingworkforceplanninghome/European workingtimedirective/index.htm (accessed 21 January 2008).

Department of Health (2008). *Raising the Profile of Long Term Conditions Care: A Compendium of Information.* London: The Stationery Office.

Dubois, C., McKee, M. & Nolte, E. (2006). *Human Resources for Health in Europe.* Milton Keynes, UK: Open University Press for the European Observatory on Health Systems and Policies; http://www.euro.who.int/Document/E87923.pdf (accessed 21 January 2008).

International Council of Nurses (2003). *Definition and Characteristics of the Role.* Geneva: International Council of Nurses; www.icn-apnetwork.org (accessed 21 January 2008).

Kay, S. (2005). *Management and Leadership: What's the Difference?* Weston, UK: Extensor; http://www.extensor.co.uk/articles/mgt_and_leadership/mgt_and_leadership.pdf (accessed 28 January 2008).

Laurant, M., Reeves, D., Hermens, R. *et al.* (2004). Substitution of doctors by nurses in primary care. *Cochrane Database of Systematic Reviews,* **4**, CD001271.

MacDonald, J. M. (2005). Higher level practice in community nursing: part two. *Nursing Standard,* **20**, 41–49.

Mantzoukas, S. & Watkinson, S. (2006). Review of advanced nursing practice: the international literature and developing the generic features. *Journal of Clinical Nursing,* **16**, 28–37.

McSherry, R. (2004). Practice development and health care governance: a recipe for modernization. *Journal of Nursing Management,* **12**, 137–146.

National Statistics (2006). Trends in health expectancies 1981–2002. *Health Statistics Quarterly,* 2006, 61–62.

NHS Modernisation Agency (2005). *10 High Impact Changes for Service Improvement and Delivery.* London: The Stationery Office.

Nightingale, S. (2007). Pilot evaluation of theatre training workshops. *Journal of Perioperative Practice*, **17**, 462–467.

Nursing and Midwifery Council (2006). *Definition of Advanced Nursing Practice*. London: Nursing and Midwifery Council; http://www.nmc-uk.org (accessed 21 January 2008).

Paterson, J. (1998). Law, ethics and risk in nursing practice. *Journal of Advanced Nursing*, **27**, 881–883.

Price, B. (2007). Professional development opportunities in changing times. *Nursing Standard*, **21**, 29–35.

QuickMBA (2008). *PEST Analysis*. http://www.quickmba.com/strategy/pest/ (accessed 23 June 2008).

Rafferty, A. M., Clarke, S., Colesm, J. *et al.* (2007). Outcomes of variation in hospital nurse staffing in English hospitals: cross-sectional analysis of survey data and discharge records. *International Journal of Nursing Studies*, **44**, 175–182.

Reid, P. (2001). A little modern magic. *Nursing Times*, **97**, 22.

Rushforth, H., Burge, D., Mullee, M. & Jones, S. (2006). Nurse-led paediatric preoperative assessment. *Paediatric Nursing*, **18**, 23–29.

Scholes, J. (2006). *Developing Expertise in Critical Care Nursing*. Oxford: Blackwell.

Wanless, D. [for HM Treasury] (2004). *Securing Good Health for the Whole Population*. London: The Stationery Office; www.hm-treasury.gov.uk/consultations_and_legislation/wanless/consult_wanless04_final.cfm (accessed 24 June 2008).

World Health Organization (2002). *Integrating Prevention into Health Care*. Geneva: World Health Organization; http://www.who.int/mediacentre/factsheets/fs172/en (accessed 21 January 2008).

World Health Organization (2006). *The World Health Report 2006: Working Together for Health*. Geneva: World Health Organization; http://www.who.int/whr/2006/en/ (accessed 21 January 2008).

10

Managing conflict in perioperative settings

Jean Hinton

Key Learning Points

- Understand the psychological origins of conflict within operating theatres
- Understand the organization contribution to conflict in theatres
- Acquire insight into techniques of conflict resolution

This chapter will discuss some of the reasons that give rise to conflict within the perioperative environment, with examples. It will then explore perceptions and assumptions and finally discuss and suggest some strategies that can aid conflict resolution.

Conflict can be described as 'A clash or struggle that occurs when a real or perceived threat or difference exists in the desires, thoughts, attitudes, feelings or behaviours of two or more parties' (Deutsch 1973; cited by Huber 2000:180). Organizational conflict can be described as the conflict that occurs when departments or factions within an organization are competing for scarce available resources. Job conflict can occur both at an individual or the organizational level where two or more people perceive opposition to goals, wishes and/or needs (Huber 2000). According to Marquis & Huston (2000), in the early twentieth century conflict was regarded as destructive and if conflict occurred it was considered to be a sign of bad management. By the middle of that century, conflict was accepted as normal but dysfunctional.

Managers were taught how to resolve conflict not how to prevent it. By the late twentieth century, managers were taught to encourage conflict as it was believed that conflict stimulated growth. However, conflict can be both good and bad and the outcomes depend on how it is managed (Cavanagh 1991, Marquis & Huston 2000).

There are three primary categories of conflict: intrapersonal, interpersonal and intergroup. Intrapersonal conflict is internal conflict where an individual is struggling within themselves over conflicting issues. Sometimes responsibilities within roles and/or their responsibilities to other members of the organization can conflict with an individual's own values and beliefs. Having the ability to cope with and resolve this conflict is vital to the mental and physical wellbeing of the individual. Interpersonal conflict occurs between two or more people or between individuals within a group or team. Intergroup conflict is a conflict occurring between two differing groups, teams, departments or organizations (Huber 2000, Marquis & Huston 2000).

Because of the nature of work carried out by healthcare professionals, which in itself can be stressful and difficult in any healthcare context, staff are more vulnerable to being exposed to, or more likely to engage in, conflict (Hipwell *et al.* 1989; cited by Vivar 2006). Therefore, managing conflict is crucial to the smooth operation of an organization, especially when effective team

Core Topics in Operating Department Practice: Leadership and Management, ed. Brian Smith, Paul Rawling, Paul Wicker and Chris Jones. Published by Cambridge University Press. © Cambridge University Press 2010.

working is essential to the health and wellbeing of the patients under its care.

Workplace conflict can be a result of different individuals or groups seeking a resolution or position that is incompatible with the wishes or needs of others. Conversely, different individuals or groups may seek to reach an agreed goal but use methods that are incompatible to the wishes or needs of others. During most people's working lives, especially in a hierarchical system, they are placed in situations where obedience is expected. However, society also expects its citizens to act according to their conscience (Hayes 1998). Conflicts of interest and beliefs do appear in the perioperative setting and can cause stress and distress for individuals.

Reflective points

- What situations have you experienced that fall into the above categories?
- How did/does it make you feel?

Although most of us think of conflict as damaging and harmful, there have been studies that have concluded that not all conflict is destructive or harmful but that in certain situations conflict can be positive and in others essential (Vivar 2006). Conflict has also been described as constructive because it can lead to new ideas, change and growth. According to Smyth (1985), 'Conflict increases creativity and innovation, provides more energy and motivation, offers people the opportunity for personal growth and healthier relationships, encourages self-examination and fosters reappraising of the situation.'

An example of conflict leading to change in the perioperative area is given in the following scenario. Two gynaecological sessions are taking place simultaneously once a week. Both sessions are consultant led. Both sessions have always had one or two patients listed for laparoscopic surgery. The theatre department only has five laparoscopic sets available, with a few extra supplementary instruments. Gradually, more and more women are being

listed for laparoscopic surgery on both sessions until up to eight or nine patients are regularly listed each week. This situation means that at least two or more patients each week are potentially going to be cancelled because of lack of instrumentation. The cancellation of less than four patients relies on some of the laparoscopic instrument sets being decontaminated and sterilized during the session, which is not always possible. This problem is leading to stressed staff, angry surgeons and distressed patients. Conflict in the form of arguments and blame is happening each week.

Common sense may tell you that more instrument sets are needed or conversely fewer patients should be selected for laparoscopic surgery each week. However, many staff may not feel empowered to do much more than complain to each other about the situation (Garland 2003). Staff may be disenchanted and frustrated with their jobs and lack self-esteem because they believe that they are undervalued within their organization (Cain 2007). Healthcare professionals do tend to make do, to squeeze everything they can out of scant resources.

How does a situation like this arise? There could be a number of reasons, for example a changeover of staff for a few weeks could mask the problem initially, with no-one realizing it is ongoing. The surgeons may not themselves select their patients nor have the relevant knowledge regarding the availability of sets. Sometimes secretaries make up the lists from criteria laid down by the surgeons: for example, one major and four minor cases to be listed. A build up of women waiting for laparoscopies would lead to more of them being listed together. Lack of communication between different departments regarding maximum number of instrument sets can result in patients being listed with no thought or forward planning relating to instrumentation. Ineffective or poor communication can cause stress and lead to conflict (Cooke 2006), as in the above scenario. The conflict in this scenario may be resolved by better communication involving all parties and by putting a business plan together to buy more instruments.

Conflict has many meanings: it can mean a clash of opposing viewpoints, a disagreement, hostility or a war. There are also different levels of conflict starting with feelings of discomfort when witnessing or being targeted in a minor disagreement rising to a crisis level if physical violence is involved.

Although perioperative staff are not presently subjected to the same amount of abuse and violence from the public as colleagues in accident and emergency (A&E) departments, there is now more contact than ever before as a result of changing boundaries and expanding roles. For example, with more stabilization bays being situated within theatre suites rather than in A&E departments, contact with patients' relatives and friends has increased for perioperative personnel. At one time, no relatives, including parents with children, were allowed through the theatre doors. This has resulted in staff having to adapt to dealing with very anxious, distressed people trying to cope with the fact that their relatives, partners or friends are gravely ill. These situations can potentially lead to anger and verbal and/or physical abuse.

Communication is the key, utilizing both verbal and non-verbal means to enable the practitioners to reassure and give clear explanations but also to recognize and understand the signals given by individuals as an indication to the possibility of potential conflict. According to Molloy & Henderson (2006:325), 'Generally, people behave according to certain well-established principles and if these principles can be recognized it can give the staff member an indication as to the likelihood of conflict taking place'.

There are many reasons for workplace conflict. These include mistakes and/or accidents, poor communication, miscommunication, misunderstanding, being judgemental, differences in values, differences in cultures, differences in goals/wants/ needs and expectations and personality clashes. Some causes of workplace conflict include competition for resources, role pressures, task interdependency, emotions, lack of clarity on who does what and lack of or non-conformance to policies and procedures regarding standards of performance. In addition, there are also the personal factors that can lead to conflict; these include self-concept, environmental factors, an individual's physical and psychological health status and an individual's past experiences (Rocchiccioli & Tilbury 1998, Huber 2000, Marquis & Houston 2000).

Multiprofessional teamwork is an essential aspect of perioperative care. Delivering high-quality, holistic patient care at an especially vulnerable time for the patients requires excellent communication skills between all the relevant professionals in addition to the knowledge, skills and dexterity to complete all aspects of the patients' perioperative experience safely. To get all the players into a theatre together at the same time (especially for emergency surgery) can feel like a minor miracle. Going back to comments above about working together for a common goal reflects this daily situation; however, whether all the players agree on a common strategy to reach their goal remains to be seen.

The surgeon believes he is in charge of the list; the anaesthetist believes the same but the team leader or designated practitioner also believes themselves to be in charge. When all is going well, the atmosphere is relaxed and all the members of the team have feelings of achievement for a job well done. Unfortunately this is not always the way things happen. The usual consultant anaesthetist is on holiday and a junior has been appointed to the theatre list. The surgeon will have expectations of working in exactly the same way as usual. In some cases no adjustments would have been made to the workload in deference to a different anaesthetist. This could be a recipe for conflict, potentially leading to a dysfunctional team. Everyone may feel under pressure and unhappy, and this situation could actually lead to patients at the end of the list being cancelled owing to lack of time. This is a lose–lose situation that could potentially have been avoided if good, effective communication had taken place. Surgeons when planning lists do not always appear to take account of the anaesthetic time. The anaesthetists do not all work at exactly the same pace or in the same way. A junior anaesthetist, for instance, will not be as quick or as confident as a consultant anaesthetist with several years more experience. This is, of course, true of any professional and this scenario could have the same outcome because the usual surgeon, scrub team or anaesthetic practitioners are on holiday or off sick.

According to Yule *et al.* (2006), the analysis of adverse events in surgery indicates that they are more likely to be caused by a breakdown in communication than technological error. Yule *et al.* (2006:1098) explain that in their medical training non-technical skills, such as leadership, are not addressed explicitly. 'However, surgeons need to demonstrate these skills, which underpin their technological excellence, to maximize patient safety in the operating theatre.' Yule *et al.* (2006) go on to state that the medical model of training focuses mainly on developing knowledge, clinical expertise and technical skills. Skills such as leadership, decision making and teamwork appear to have to be developed informally.

Perceptions

Perceptions are based on our personal experiences in life, which means that how we interpret present-day events is based on what we have experienced in past events (Gregory; cited by Hayes 1998).

It is important to remember that what others feel, see and/or experience is true and real to them regardless of how we ourselves feel. Most people will initially perceive an event somewhat differently. Valentine (2001), in an article on gender perspective on conflict, reports on studies into gender differences in approaches to conflict. She comments that the studies demonstrated that men and women perceived and dealt with conflict differently. Women tend to be more empathetic and would be more likely to deal with conflict through negotiation and/or mediation while men will try persuasion and influence.

What would you believe in the following scenario? A fellow team member had become more and more withdrawn over the past few months.

Most days she acted normally but you had noticed that more often there were days when she almost ignored everyone, appearing preoccupied. Lately, the situation appeared to be getting much worse. Her attendance had become somewhat erratic as had her mood swings and concentration span. Other members of the team were beginning to complain about having to work with the individual as everyone felt she was not functioning to the best of her ability and that she was becoming a liability to herself and others. Rumours abounded that she had arrived for work more than once with what appeared to be the effects of a hangover, looking scruffy and tired. An attempt by her friends and colleagues to speak to her had led to an angry exchange of words, which had basically isolated her from everyone in the team. The whole team became stressed, arguments escalated and the high standard of work declined; mistakes occurred more often.

The above is fabricated but consider the situation for a few minutes. What do you believe to be the problem? Has she got a drink problem? Has she got money worries? Could she be in an abusive relationship? Is she ill or is someone close to her ill or possibly dying?

The truth is that the problem could be any of the above or maybe something totally different. The hard part is that not knowing the facts we would all interpret the situation to make sense of what we believe, observe or feel ourselves (Hayes 1998). Valentine *et al.* (1997) highlight the fact that conflict, in a team context, can break down personal and work relationships, which, in turn, can lead to the rejection of a team member or members, as in the above scenario, and has the potential to culminate in not meeting individual or team goals or even in violence.

If the team member had confided in her colleagues, the situation would have developed differently; some of her team colleagues would perhaps have been empathetic while others may have offered practical suggestions. It may still have been a difficult and emotional time for all but such extreme conflict and stress may have been avoided. De Drue *et al.* (2001:200) state that emotions arise when concerns are expressed and that they are not just an internal state of mind but 'processes that develop both within and between individuals'. For instance, in the team context, if words are spoken between two individuals no overt anger may be evident; however, if other team members are present their reaction may provoke anger and confrontation between the two individuals.

What changes perceptions?

Jormsri (2004) highlights the moral issues regarding patient care. He talks about patient care as being a many faceted phenomenon requiring the knowledge and skills of the multiprofessional team. This phenomenon according to Jormsri (2004) requires all the professionals to respect each other's values, beliefs and responsibilities. Moral conflict can occur if those values, beliefs and opinions are totally opposed.

Perceptions, assumptions and opinions can be changed by incorporating new or additional information into a situation, as described above. Another way is a paradigm shift. A paradigm is a set of assumptions, concepts, values and practices that belong to the community that shares them (Kuhn 1962; cited by Haralambos & Holborn 2000). A paradigm shift, therefore, describes a basic change in the above assumptions.

Understanding another person's perceptions can change your own perceptions, or at least aid in finding solutions. If you perceive the other person's goals as compatible with your own, you are more likely to engage in constructive open-minded debate about each other's views, values and beliefs. If, however, you perceive others' goals to be incompatible with your own, you are more likely to avoid debate, become aggressive and/or undermine each others decisions (Almost 2006).

Assumptions

Learn to assume nothing; things are rarely as they seem. Ask questions as it is harder to be wrong if you ask first. Always try to understand the other person's perspective before you try to get him or her to understand yours. If someone appears to be acting irrationally, consider alternative reasons for that behaviour, do not just take it at face value.

During any situation where conflict arises it is important to try to avoid becoming defensive. Always allow the other person(s) to verbalize their experience(s) and perception(s) of the given situation. Sometimes the thing we believe is the solution could be part of the problem. According to Field & Nolan (2004), work done during the Northern Ireland conflict demonstrates that people must be allowed to tell their own story as they wish, be believed by others and then take responsibility for their actions if conflict is ever to be resolved.

It is important during any conflict to remember that the goal is to listen, not to be right. When the other person is talking, listen actively; do not spend the time trying to formulate your reply. Always reiterate and repeat what is being said to make sure you did understand and to reassure the other person that you were actually listening to what they were saying.

Problem-solving skills

Always focus on the actual problem. Try to avoid thinking about or bringing up issues that happened in the past. In other words, try not to personalize or get emotional; focus instead on the facts of the problem and strive to identify possible solutions. Two or more brains can potentially generate more ideas and possible solutions, so where relevant mind map, discuss and analyse the problem and empower staff to have some influence and control when dealing with problems. Giving ownership to others can also be helpful when instigating any changes required in solving the problem. Problem solving carried out under restrictions or by one individual can deny an organization or department the benefits of utilizing collective staff knowledge and skills and encouraging group cohesion.

Janis & Mann (1977; cited by Cox & Thompson 2000) viewed problem solving as an opportunity for both individuals and groups to be creative while demonstrating both their professional judgement and competence.

Always remember that when a solution is agreed upon and put in place, evaluation of its effectiveness is crucial. All healthcare personnel are used to continually checking and evaluating the progress of patients under their care. This is to enable reaction to any deviations in their health that occur and possibly to anticipate and treat any potential problems before they happen or become worse. This maxim applies to all situations. Just because the solution devised is believed to be the best solution to a problem, it does not mean that some flexibility may not be required. It may also be the case that a good solution one day may not be so good the next, particularly within the constantly changing and adapting world of the NHS.

Different strategies for dealing with conflict

According to Bar-Tal (2000:354), 'conflict resolution refers to a political process through which the parties in conflict eliminate the perceived incompatibility between their goals and interests and establish a new situation of perceived compatibility'.

There are five common strategies used to resolve conflict (Vivar 2006). They are:

avoidance: 'Conflict, what conflict?'
accommodating: 'What ever you say is OK with me'
competition: 'My way or else'
collaboration: 'How can we work together to solve this problem?'
compromise: 'Shall we split the difference'.

How a person resolves a conflict may depend on what personality type they are. People have differing styles when dealing with conflict. Some people will mentally and physically withdraw from any kind of conflict, while others will postpone any potential confrontation. Some people will sit on the fence and will neither agree nor disagree in a conflict issue, while others become very aggressive and argumentative. There are others who will not explicitly show their disagreement but will be covert using gossip or sabotage to undermine the wishes and/or actions of others. Being aware of your own style and the fact that others have differing styles may help to manage a positive outcome to a conflict situation effectively (Huber 2000, Tomey 2000).

There are various sources of potential conflict within the healthcare environment, including badly communicated or unexplained management decisions or actions, lack of trust of the management team and/or of co-workers, staffing levels and workload and staff perspectives resulting in high stress levels, low morale and a disenchanted, frustrated workforce (Almost 2006, Vivar 2006).

It is important to deal with conflict as soon as possible as leaving it to fester or grow will exacerbate any situation. If the conflict is in groups, then the solution may be found within the group. A group discussion can sometimes open up the opportunity to resolve conflict by reaching an understanding or clearing up a misunderstanding or miscommunication.

Example scenario of dealing with conflict

In the following scenario consider which of the five common conflict resolution strategies you believe to be the most appropriate. Justify your choice and give reasons for rejecting the others.

You have been qualified for 18 months working on a rotational basis in the operating theatres of a busy district general hospital situated close to several busy 'A' roads and motorways. You are gaining experience and are well thought of and have recently been given more responsibility. You have also been asked to deputize for the team leader on a few occasions. Your anaesthetic experience is varied to enable you to work out of hours on-call. Your scrub experience since qualifying has mainly been within the general, gynaecological and urological surgery teams. You have just moved into the orthopaedic trauma theatre team for scrub and are on your second week. The last time you did orthopaedic scrub was over two years ago as a student. You arrive on duty to find that influenza has caused excessive sickness and that you are in charge of the trauma list. The staff you have been allocated are one other scrub nurse from the ENT scrub team and an experienced orthopaedic support worker. On the trauma list is a patient with polytrauma who needs quite extensive surgery. You protest to the theatre coordinator that you do not have sufficient knowledge or experience regarding the procedure, equipment or surgeon and have no experienced scrub staff to help you. The theatre coordinator replies that owing to the staff shortages you will just have to do the best you can. What should you do? You will have to decide between your professional, personal and organizational obligations.

Discussion of conflict resolution options

You need to consider your position, the theatre coordinator's position and a position on which you can both agree. Your position is that you want to do your best for the patient, the medical team and not contravene your Code of Conduct (Health Professions Council 2008, Nursing and Midwifery Council 2008). The coordinator's position is that he or she is trying to provide a service for everyone without having to cancel lists and distress the patients. A mutually compatible position could be that neither of you want to do anything that could potentially bring risk or harm to a patient, yourselves or your organization.

Look at the following strategies for conflict resolution.

Accommodating. Would you really consider this choice? As you are inexperienced in this speciality then you are unqualified to run this list without other relevantly, experienced staff present. You are putting your patient, yourself, your coordinator and your careers at risk. This does not meet your mutually compatible position.

Avoiding. This is a problem that needs a quick solution and so it is not possible to avoid the problem.

Compromising. You could possibly negotiate a solution if there is a suitably experienced orthopaedic scrub practitioner you could swap with or to swap the ENT scrub practitioner with. Or you could possibly call on staff from a sister hospital within the Trust or a different theatre suite within the hospital. This compromise could possibly meet your mutually compatible position.

Collaborating. Discussing with your theatre coordinator the possible repercussions of placing an inexperienced practitioner in this position could achieve a joint effort to resolve this situation safely. This relies on the senior member of staff having the time and inclination to listen to his or her junior staff member.

Competing. Sometimes competing is the only recourse open to you in resolving conflict. It means someone has to win or lose and in this situation it could lead to complaints of you being uncooperative or insubordinate. You have to be honest and ask yourself if you are really not qualified or experienced enough to do this list. If you still feel unqualified then you would have to try and adopt an assertive approach. You could say 'I cannot run this list as I feel that I would not be able to give an appropriate service to the surgeon(s) and this could possibly result in the patient being put at risk'. It would then be very difficult for the theatre coordinator to enforce his or her allocation of you.

Remember that aggressive behaviour leads to a win–lose situation where a person may be loud and threatening, needing to be controlling and wanting to deny the rights of others.

Passive behaviour leads to a lose–win situation where you deny your own rights, fail to express an opinion and avoid eye contact with others. Assertive behaviour by comparison leads to a win–win situation where you acknowledge your own and other's rights; you are willing to compromise, and you conduct yourself in a polite, persistent manner (Huber 2000, Tomey 2000).

Conflict solution versus conflict management

Higgerson (1996) discusses the difference between conflict solution and conflict management. Conflict resolution aims to eradicate all aspects of the conflict. Attempts to resolve conflict may require outcomes that realistically may be unattainable or even undesirable to the individual, the team or the organization. Conflict management, by comparison, acknowledges that everyone has different beliefs, values and attitudes and perceives the same situations differently. Conflict management can be utilized in a positive way to create an innovative and productive workforce. A healthy work environment welcomes disagreement, discussion and debate as a possible way of reaching a mutually agreed positive outcome (Higgerson 1996).

Communication strategies

When dealing with any type of conflict, communication is the key. Personality clashes are common in all departments and can be managed using good communication skills and sensitivity. Always be clear in what is said and how it is said. Do not hint, be direct. Use 'I' statements and do not be vague; utilize good listening and answering techniques and reframe and validate the discussion contents. Make sure everyone involved understands and are all talking about the same thing.

When is conflict over?

Marquis & Huston (2000:363) state that 'consensus is always an appropriate goal in resolving conflicts and in negotiation'. Therefore, if the physical wellbeing and feelings of self-worth of all the relevant parties are preserved, in addition to a willingness of the parties to agree one option where other options were available, then the conflict is over. According to Marquis & Huston (2000), the biggest challenge in resolving conflict through consensus is that it takes time and requires all parties to be good communicators, flexible and open minded.

REFERENCES

Almost, J. (2006). Conflict within nursing work environments: concept analysis. *Journal of Advanced Nursing*, **53**, 444–453.

Bar-Tal, D. (2000). From intractable conflict through conflict resolution to reconciliation: psychological analysis. *Political Psychology*, **21**, 351–365.

Cain, J. (2007). My experience of a business course leader: a personal reflection. *Journal of Perioperative Practice*, **17**, 12–15.

Cavanagh, S.J. (1991). The conflict management style of staff nurses and nurse managers. *Journal of Advanced Nursing*, **16**, 1254–1260.

Cooke, L. (2006). Conflict and challenging behaviour in the workplace. *Journal of Perioperative Practice*, **16**, 365–366.

Cox, T. & Thomson, L. (2000). Organisational healthiness, work related stress and employee health. In Dewe, P., Leiter, M.P. & Cox, T. (eds.) *Coping, Health and Organisations*, pp. 177–194. London: Taylor & Francis.

De Drue, C.K.W., West, M.A., Fischer, A.H. & MacCurtain, S. (2001). Origins and consequences of emotions in organisational teams. In Payne, R.L. & Cooper, C.L. (eds.) *Emotions at Work: Theory, Research and Applications for Management*, pp. 199–217. Chichester, UK: John Wiley.

Field, H. & Nolan, P. (2004). What lessons can we learn from conflict resolution? *British Journal of Nursing*, **13**, 237.

Garland, G. (2003). Building on the success of LEO. *Nursing Management, RCNP,* **10**, 16–18.

Haralambos, M. & Holborn, M. (2000). *Sociology Themes and Perspectives*, 5th edn. London: Harper Collins.

Hayes, N. (1998). *Foundations of Psychology: An Introductory Text*. Walton-on-Thames, UK: Thomas Nelson.

Health Professions Council (2008). *Standards of Conduct, Performance and Ethics*. London: Health Professions Council.

Higgerson, M.L. (1996). *Communication Skills for Department Chairs*. Bolton, MA: Anker.

Huber, D. (2000). *Leadership and Nursing Care Management*. Philadelphia, PA: Saunders.

Jormsri, P. (2004). Moral conflict and collaborative mode as moral conflict resolution in health care. *Nursing and Health Services*, **6**, 217–221.

Marquis, B.L. & Huston, C.J. (2000). *Leadership Roles and Management Functions in Nursing: Theory and Application*. Philadelphia, PA: Lippincott Williams & Wilkins.

Molloy, S. & Henderson, I. (2006). Conflict resolution training in the NHS. *Journal of Perioperative Practice*, **16**, 323–326.

Nursing and Midwifery Council (2008). *Code of Professional Conduct: Standards for Conduct, Performance and Ethics*. London: Nursing and Midwifery Council.

Rocchiccioli, J.T. & Tilbury, M.S. (1998). *Clinical Leadership in Nursing*. Philadelphia, PA: Saunders.

Smyth T. (1985). Management: confronting conflict. *Nursing Mirror*, **160**, 23–25.

Tomey, A.M. (2000). *Guide to Nursing Management and Leadership*, 6th edn. St Louis, MI: Mosby.

Valentine, P.E.B. (2001). A gender perspective on conflict management strategies of nurses. *Journal of Nursing Scholarship*, **33**, 69–74.

Valentine, P.E.B., Richardson, S., Wood, M. & Godkin, D. (1997). In conflict with conflict. *Canadian Journal of Nursing Administration*, **10**, 23–44.

Vivar, C.G. (2006). Putting conflict management into practice: a nursing case study. *Journal of Nursing Management*, **14**, 201–206.

Yule, S., Fun, R., Paterson-Brown, S., Maran, N. & Rowley, D. (2006). Development of a rating system for surgeons' non-technical skills. *Medical Education*, **40**, 1098–1104.

11

The management and organization of emergency operating lists

Lee Bennett

Key Learning Points

- Understand the problem of emergency perioperative provision in NHS trusts
- Consider the material and human resources required to deliver efficient emergency perioperative care
- Outline the political and professional drivers of change in emergency surgical services
- Understand the impact of unexpected events such as major civilian incidents on the rest of the surgical service

Introduction

The management and organization of the emergency operating list is not a static process but a constant process of assessment and priority management. This chapter aims to provide some insight into the organization, management and leadership of such a surgical list.

Prior to the introduction into the NHS of dedicated emergency operating rooms, urgent surgical procedures were commonly left until the end of elective lists. Most of these operations were usually performed by junior grade surgeons without the supervision of an experienced consultant, with the majority of cases being performed out of hours (Wyatt *et al.* 1990). *The Report of a Confidential Enquiry into Perioperative Deaths* (CEPOD; Buck *et al.* 1987) clearly demonstrated the need for increased supervision of junior surgeons. In

response to the publication of this paper, many NHS Trusts went on to provide dedicated emergency surgical operating rooms.

Management of these emergency surgical lists is an area that requires a great deal of communication between the multidisciplinary team (National Confidential Enquiry into Patient Outcome and Death 2007).

Definition of an emergency patient

The definition for an emergency patient is taken from the CEPOD report (Buck *et al.* 1987), which groups emergency patients into two clear categories:

emergency: immediate operation usually within one hour of surgical consultation, usually lifesaving, resuscitation carried out simultaneously with surgical treatment

urgent: operation required as soon as possible after resuscitation, usually within 24 hours of the surgical consultation.

Patients who are booked on the emergency list and are classified as urgent will have surgery prioritized according to the availability of the surgical team and the length of time waiting for surgery. When a patient with an emergency classification is added to the list, then that patient takes clinical priority over

Core Topics in Operating Department Practice: Leadership and Management, ed. Brian Smith, Paul Rawling, Paul Wicker and Chris Jones. Published by Cambridge University Press. © Cambridge University Press 2010.

the other urgent patients. A surgical team wishing to interrupt the list should be advised to communicate with the other surgical teams whose patients are waiting surgery. An emergency coordinator may be useful at this point to ensure that the most effective use is made of operating room time and resources.

To help to reduce the incidence of out-of-hours operating on urgent patients, many Trusts now operate a trauma/semi-urgent list where patients have their operations during working hours. The Royal College of Surgeons of Edinburgh (1998) state that the use of such lists leads to 80% of urgent cases being performed in normal working hours. These lists should not contain elective patients and have a perioperative team available to take urgent patients from the emergency list, allowing them to undergo their surgery in normal hours while freeing up the emergency list for emergency patients.

Many Trusts also operate a 9-to-5 urgent trauma list where patients with orthopaedic injuries are cared for. So, from the point of view of management, it is of paramount importance to have two operating rooms for urgent or emergency patients, each having a coordinator with communication between the two.

Utilization of these lists also depends on the availability of other members of the team, including radiographers and other allied health professionals, and the availability of surgical equipment.

According to *Who Operates When I* and *II* (National Confidential Enquiry into Patient Outcome and Death 1997, 2003), in an ideal world hospitals that admit emergency trauma victims should have a dedicated trauma list daily, and those that admit surgical emergencies should also have a dedicated operating room that is funded for anaesthetic and surgical cover and have the appropriate skill mix of nursing and allied health professionals.

Staffing

Adequate skill mix for the staffing of emergency operating rooms is suggested by several leading bodies. The *Standards and Recommendations for Safe Perioperative Practice* (Association for Perioperative Practice 2007) defines the minimum recommended numbers and skill mix of the practitioners. These guidelines suggest the following Association for Perioperative Practice (2007:121):

- one qualified anaesthetic assistant practitioner for each session involving an anaesthetic
- two qualified scrub practitioners
- one appropriately trained circulating person
- two trained circulating practitioners where the operative procedure involves two cavities being opened simultaneously and has two operating teams at the operating table
- one appropriately trained recovery practitioner to care for the patient; there may be occasions where two qualified practitioners are required if there is a quick throughput of patients requiring minor procedures such as in the surgical day unit.

The Association of Anaesthetists of Great Britain and Ireland (2003) suggest the use of senior anaesthetists and surgeons when staffing the emergency operating room. Overall management of the list and coordination should occur with a senior practitioner undertaking the role of emergency surgical coordinator. The coordinator is responsible for the management of the operating list and should work alongside the senior medical staff in the emergency operating room, communicating with the perioperative team and coordinating the booking of patients for surgery. The role of emergency surgical coordinator is crucial for ensuring the list runs smoothly and so should be carried out by a senior practitioner with experience of the area and a defined job description.

Skill mix is important for staffing the emergency operating list and it is important to consider the level of experience and qualification of the team working in the emergency operating room. Commitments outside the operating department also need to be taken into consideration. For example the operating department practitioner providing anaesthetic support services may be required to attend cardiac arrest calls, trauma calls, emergencies in the accident and emergency (A&E) department or give assistance on the ward. If the hospital receives trauma patients, assessing the most appropriate skill mix is vital in out-of-hours emergencies because of the wide range of surgical problems that the patient may present with.

It is the responsibility of the surgical coordinator to ensure that there is an appropriate skill mix in order for the service to work efficiently. With perioperative practitioners who are able to take on more than one clinical role, the coordinator may have the availability and flexibility to change them around according to the surgical requirements and the practitioner's experience.

It is important that the coordinator maintains overall responsibility for the coordination and the management of the list; however, there may be occasions when the department gets so busy that the coordinator may have to become involved in clinical practice. This should be avoided wherever possible given that the busier the department is then the more need there is for the coordinator to maintain control and provide direction for the team. A coordinator cannot coordinate if he or she is taken up with scrubbing for a procedure. If this happens on more than the occasional basis, it needs to be addressed by senior management to ensure that the skill mix and staffing levels are appropriate for the level of work carried out in the department.

There is also the risk that practitioners who only work on emergency lists might lose their clinical skills in specialist areas that only have operating lists during normal working hours. A solution carried out in some Trusts is to rotate practitioners around the clinical areas to ensure that clinical skills are not lost.

The role of the emergency surgical coordinator

The role of the surgical coordinator is predominately that of a leader, having the responsibility of controlling, directing and supporting the progression of the operating list. Depending on experience and grade, this role may be allocated to the senior scrub practitioner or, in some cases, the anaesthetic practitioner. The coordinator is responsible for the booking, sending and overall care of the patient in the emergency operating room. Good leadership skills are required, with the practitioner undertaking a mainly non-clinical role.

Although assessing clinical need and priority is mainly a medical decision, the coordinator will have a large input into the prioritization of the list in order to ensure that resources are used efficiently. The coordinator must have excellent communication skills and the ability to delegate tasks to members of the team. The coordinator may also be able to mediate discussions between the medical staff when, for example, there are disagreements over which case has priority.

The coordinator should possess excellent organizational skills and have the experience required to be able to provide support and expert advice when required to every member of the emergency team. The ability to control the list is of paramount importance when it comes to fasting of patients which is discussed further in this chapter.

The surgical coordinator has the overall management and responsibility for the non-medical staff who are working in the emergency operating room and also has a large input into the organization of the operating list, although overall clinical responsibility will be held by the consultant anaesthetist who is allocated to the emergency/trauma operating room. At times of stress, it is important that all members of the team have input into the decision making. For example, it would be wasteful if the anaesthetist sent for a patient before any anaesthetic assistance was available, regardless of the urgency of the case. Similarly, an orthopaedic surgeon insisting that his or her case needed to go first would be well advised to check that specialist equipment was available first. This juggling of priorities, negotiating with surgeons, anaesthetists, perioperative practitioners, ward staff and others, and understanding of resource implications are the most valuable skills that the coordinator needs.

A clearly defined role for the emergency coordinator should be developed to minimize misunderstandings and to optimize the surgical time on the emergency operating list. The coordinator has to ensure that the perioperative team are suitably refreshed and have adequate support during their clinical work. In situations where there is a traumatic event, such as death during surgery, the coordinator may need to arrange for counselling or support for practitioners.

The role of the coordinator is a challenging role that requires high levels of knowledge and experience, and excellent skills in communication, management and delegation.

Booking patients

The booking of patients for surgery requires good communication between the admitting surgical team, the perioperative team and the nurses on the wards. The surgical team should book patients and discuss the patient's condition with the anaesthetist to minimize risks during surgery. Time should be allowed for the anaesthetist to assess the patient preoperatively (Association of Anaesthetists of Great Britain and Ireland 2003).

The surgical team must be aware of fasting times and clinical priority when rapid sequence induction and ventilation are required for acutely ill patients. Anecdotal evidence suggests that delays in operating department admission are often caused by patients not being prepared for surgery appropriately. It is the responsibility of the admitting surgical team to ensure that the patient is ready for surgery and that all investigations and clinical tests have been booked with the appropriate laboratory.

Sometimes surgeons will ask for a specific time for booking the patient on to the operating list because they have other commitments, such as clinics. It is normally important not to book emergency patients for specific times as delays can occur because of equipment failure, inadequate staffing levels and in preparing the patient for surgery.

Again, communication is paramount between all specialties and the operating department. Prior to requesting the patient to be brought to the operating room from the ward, the coordinator should ensure that the patient has been fully prepared for surgery.

Emergencies sent directly to the operating room

There may be some occasions when seriously ill patients are transferred directly to the operating room (Box 11.1) and surgery and resuscitation will run concurrently. When this happens, the coordinator needs to be aware of the need to carefully integrate all the members of the team to ensure the patient receives optimal care. There may have been no time to organize tests or investigations such as transfusion status, consent status and starvation times. Here good communication is particularly important to ensure that important tests or investigations are carried out prior to surgery.

Excessive bleeding, rupture of great vessels, severe limb trauma and, in paediatrics, torsion of the testis, require a patient to be brought directly to the operating room to ensure there is minimal delay for surgery.

In cases such as this, the coordinator needs to show their leadership and people management skills to ensure that the operating room is ready and the perioperative team are allocated tasks to ensure safe and optimal care for the patient.

Box 11.1 Situations requiring direct transfer to the operating room

Aortic aneurysm (adults)

Torsion of testis (paediatrics)

Pulse-less fracture

Patients that require urgent surgical intervention for bleeding while undergoing fluid resuscitation or cardiopulmonary resuscitation

Patients with neurological conditions with a reduced level of consciousness, for example a blocked shunt with raised intracranial pressures

Patients with time critical heart conditions, for example cardiac tamponade

---

Patient fasting

Managing the fasting times of patients can be a demanding process in itself. The admission of emergency patients to the operating list, change of surgeons, availability of surgical sundries along with delays in getting patients to the operating department can all increase the length of fasting times in all categories of patient.

In the document *Preoperative Assessment and the Role of the Anaesthetist* published by the Association of Anaesthetists of Great Britain and Ireland (2001), it clearly states that the risk of aspiration of the contents of the stomach into the lungs should be minimized by ensuring that patients do not eat or drink prior to anaesthesia and surgery. The document goes on to suggest that patients should undergo the following fasting times in accordance with guidance taken from the American Association of Anaesthesiologists:

- solid food, infant formula or other milk: 6 hours
- breast milk: 4 hours
- clear fluid (non-carbonated): 2 hours.

These times may need to be waived for emergency patients requiring urgent surgery. Such cases require careful balancing of the risks and where required guidance should be sought from medical staff. When fasting has not occurred, the use of rapid-sequence induction of anaesthesia with cricoid pressure is recommended.

The Association of Anaesthetists of Great Britain and Ireland (2001) go on to suggest that patients who have undergone bowel preparation, pregnant mothers, sick patients and children should not be fasted for long periods of time without consideration of their hydration needs.

Where patients have been admitted to the operating department and have been waiting for a long time, they may need rehydrating with oral clear fluids, if they can be tolerated, for up to two hours prior to surgery, or intravenous fluids prescribed by the anaesthetist, to prevent dehydration of the patient prior to surgery.

Although it is in the best interests of the patient, care should be taken when giving patients fluids to drink as this may cause a delay in the patient having surgery if other patients are cancelled on the emergency list. Close liaison should occur with the anaesthetist on the emergency list prior to giving patients drinks.

Particular care is required for patients with diabetes. If possible, such patients should have their surgery at the earliest opportunity in order to maintain their blood sugar levels. Patients may require intravenous fluids and dextrose in order to control their blood sugar levels.

Local policies and protocols should be drawn up in conjunction with the anaesthetic department to reduce misunderstandings and to ensure that the risks to the patient are minimized.

Clinical priorities

Assessing the clinical priority of patients requiring surgery is an ongoing process between the surgical and anaesthetic staff and can often be observed as a constant fight between surgical specialties in order to get their patients treated first. It is common, for example, for surgeons with patients with acute abdominal symptoms to try and prioritize their patients before those of an orthopaedic surgeon with elderly patients with fractured necks of femurs. Clinical priorities are a medical matter and the practitioner should be careful not to be pulled into the discussion. However, even in these discussions, the coordinator can help the medical staff to make their decisions based on resources, such as equipment and staff, which are available. Commonly, patients on the emergency list are operated on in accordance with the time at which they were booked. In cases where the medical staff feel that their patient requires surgery sooner than anticipated, then they should liaise in the first instance with the anaesthetist and coordinator in order to identify patients needs and then agree with the other surgeons to move their patient forward on the list. Only if all other specialities are in agreement may the surgeon do this.

Major incident

The management of a major incident is a vast and complex event that requires multilevel communication not only in a single department but across the hospital and in many situations outside the hospital too. Dedicated texts have been produced in order to define major incidents. The Advanced Life Support Group (2003) defines a major incident as a need for 'special or extraordinary arrangements' needed for services to cope.

A major incident is usually triggered by one of the emergency services if the incident is external or by the hospital if there is an internal emergency. The NHS Trusts have devised plans in order to cope with major incidents and practitioners must be aware of these.

Most NHS Trusts also have local plans drawn up in case of a major incident being declared that consider how to deal with the incident and how to deal with the impact that this may have on both emergency and elective surgery. If the incident is declared as a medical incident, then the impact on surgery may well be lower. Assistance may be required for airway assessment and management in the A&E department. If the incident is a surgical/trauma incident, then the demand for surgery will increase.

When the incident is a surgical crisis, practitioners may need to be sent to the A&E department (primarily anaesthetic support staff) for the resuscitation of patients. Elective surgery may have to be delayed in order to free operating rooms for the immediate surgery of patients suffering from pulse-less limbs, cardiothoracic trauma or neurological insult.

Patients listed for elective procedures may be cancelled to free up surgical beds when there are high numbers of patients likely to be admitted to the hospital following a major incident. Careful management may be needed to avoid the A&E department becoming overcrowded with staff.

The following items relating to the management of a major incident are important when drawing up plans:

- job roles of staff groups relevant to a major incident
- communication link with the A&E department and the emergency operating department coordinator
- formulation of a role for the most senior member of staff to coordinate the operating department activities especially in the event of an out-of-hours emergency
- call-in policy for perioperative practitioners
- a representative of the operating department staff to attend hospital planning meetings
- cancellation of patients.

This is not an exhaustive list but hopefully gives an insight into the key points surrounding major incident management. Further reading should be taken from dedicated books and literature relevant to the planning and management of a major incident. During a major incident, communication is the key factor that defines the running of a smooth operation.

REFERENCES

Advanced Life Support Group (2003). *Major Incident Medical Management and Support: The Practical Approach*. London: BMJ Publishing.

Association for Perioperative Practice (2007). *Standards and Recommendations for Safe Perioperative Practice*. Harrogate: Association for Perioperative Practice.

Association of Anaesthetists of Great Britain and Ireland (2001). *Preoperative Assessment and the Role of the Anaesthetist*. London: Association of Anaesthetists of Great Britain and Ireland.

Association of Anaesthetists of Great Britain and Ireland (2003). *Theatre Efficiency, Safety, Quality of Care and Optimal Use of Resources*. London: Association of Anaesthetists of Great Britain and Ireland.

Buck, N., Devlin, H.B. & Lunn, J.N.D. (1987). *Report of the Confidential Enquiry into Perioperative Deaths*. London: Nuffield Provincial Hospital Trusts and The King's Fund.

National Confidential Enquiry into Patient Outcome and Death (1997). *Who Operates When? The 1997 Report of the National Confidential Enquiry into Perioperative Deaths 1996/1997*. Bristol: National Confidential Enquiry into Patient Outcome and Death.

National Confidential Enquiry into Patient Outcome and Death (2003). *Who Operates When? II. The 2003 Report of the National Confidential Enquiry into Perioperative Deaths.* Bristol: National Confidential Enquiry into Patient Outcome and Death.

National Confidential Enquiry into Patient Outcome and Death (2007). *Trauma: Who Cares?* London: National Confidential Enquiry into Patient Outcome and Death.

Royal College of Surgeons of Edinburgh (1998). The effect of a dedicated theatre facility on emergency operating patterns. *Journal of the Royal College of Surgeons of Edinburgh*, **43**, 17–19.

Wyatt, M.G., Houghton, P.W. & Brodribb, A.J. (1990). Theatre delay for emergency general surgery patients; a cause for concern? *Annals of the Royal College of Surgeons of England*, **72**, 236–238.

12

Organizational culture

Charlotte Moen

Key Learning Points

- Identify the issues relating to 'culture' within an organization and team
- Understand how the concept of culture can be applied to an organization and team
- Understand the unwritten rules
- Understand how culture can be influenced
- Develop self-awareness within a leadership role

Introduction

There are several keys to successful leadership. One is an understanding of the critical role culture plays, particularly when implementing change and promoting innovation. Another is an awareness of how culture can be manipulated to promote a more effective and receptive learning environment. However, cultural manipulation is not easy. Furthermore, the concept is hard to define, analyse and measure (Schein 1997). The aim of this chapter is to challenge personal views about culture within both the organization and the team; uncover some of the unwritten rules; reflect on the links between culture, change management and leadership; and provide some tips for success and for empowering the development of effective leadership skills. To support the translation of theory to practice, a reflective model to aid cultural awareness will be proposed.

Throughout the chapter, reflection points have been included to aid self-awareness. The information in the boxes will allow reflection on the context of the text in terms of personal experience and position on the leadership learning continuum.

What do we mean by culture?

Defining culture is not as easy as may be thought (Handy 1993). So a clear understanding of what culture means seems an appropriate place to start. Ask any healthcare worker about culture and everyone agrees it exists; often it is apparent that there are different subcultures operating at different levels of an organization, in different professional groups and also in different wards, departments, clinics, theatres, GP surgeries and so on. Issues of culture are not just pertinent to healthcare but affect any organization (Handy 1993). It is also recognized that having the right culture is vital for the successful implementation of change, for the performance of individuals and teams, and for quality and patient safety. However, ask anyone to define what they mean by culture and you are met with silence. Culture has been defined in several ways:

- 'Something that is perceived, something felt' (Handy 1993:191)
- 'Sets of values and norms and beliefs – reflected in different structures and systems' (Handy 1993:180)

Core Topics in Operating Department Practice: Leadership and Management, ed. Brian Smith, Paul Rawling, Paul Wicker and Chris Jones. Published by Cambridge University Press. © Cambridge University Press 2010.

- 'A pattern of shared basic assumptions that the group has learned as it solved its problems . . . the way to perceive, think and feel in relation to those problems' (Schein 1997:12)
- 'Prevailing values and ethos of a particular nation' (Vincent 2006).

Can these definitions be applied to a health service? They can in that culture implies shared values, assumptions and beliefs, which are generally deeply embedded and affect the behaviour of staff. Hardacre (2001:32) defines health culture as the 'values and beliefs espoused by the organization' or 'the way we do things around here'. Sullivan & Decker (2005) discuss culture in terms of 'the norms and traditions' of the organization and Handy (1993) adds that customs and traditions are a powerful influence on behaviour. This is particularly true in health where many aspects of care are ritualistic and are not challenged, partly because of the hierarchical nature of the NHS and partly because of the difficulties associated with implementing change. So a definition of culture in relation to health must encompass the concept of ritualistic practice and reflect the need to decipher a 'secret code' of rules that allows staff to understand the expected patterns of behaviour and ways of working. Culture also encompasses the organization's past successes, philosophy, goals, standards and attitudes (Palmer 2001). So to understand the concept of culture, the following must be considered (Institute for Innovation and Improvement 2005):

- culture is about how things are done within a workplace
- culture is the way things are done within a team and is heavily influenced by shared unwritten rules
- culture reflects what has worked well in the past.

In other words it is about how people make judgements and whether they are receptive to change; it determines how people behave, what they say and how they say it and it impacts on how people work together under normal working conditions and in a crisis. Culture is, therefore, embedded into every level of the organization and its influence should not be underestimated (Faugier & Woolnough 2002).

Reflective points

- What set of values, beliefs and styles of behaviour characterize your organization and your team? Are the two sets similar? If not, why not?
- Do operating theatre staff need to generate anything special in the way of culture? If so what?
- Do theatre staff regard themselves as fully integrated into hospital life or rather set apart from the main hospital culture?

Describing organizational culture

There are various methods to categorize culture. Palmer (2001) describes two types of culture: formal and informal. Formal culture is what can be seen and measured, for example the organization's philosophy of care, objectives, annual prospectus, strategy, policy for handling complaints or patient safety incidents. Informal culture is the way the culture operates and this may differ from the formal culture an organization believes or would like to believe is in place. Examples include accepted values, beliefs and behaviour; attitudes towards sickness; dress code; dealing with conflict; implementing change; acceptable practices, such as when is late considered late – 5 minutes, 10 minutes, half an hour? Palmer (2001) argues that informal culture is based on reality and this supports the previous definition of 'the way things are done around here' (Hardacre 2001:32). Senior & Fleming (2006:138) describe formal culture as the 'more easy-to-see' and formal aspects of an organization, where the focus is on goals and objectives. By comparison, informal culture is 'hidden . . . composed of the more covert aspects of organizational life' and these norms of behaviour are rarely articulated or discussed. The largest influence is the informal culture (Senior & Fleming 2006) and it is this that drives and, it could be argued, determines the outcomes of the decision-making process and dictates whether changes are successful.

Handy (1993) defines four types of culture – power, role, task and person – and discusses a descriptor for each type to illustrate his ideas. In a 'power culture', the power is held by an individual or a small group of individuals (the analogy is a spider in the middle controlling what happens) whereas in 'role culture' the power is hierarchical and determined by position (like a Greek temple representing logic, rules and regulations). In 'task culture', the focus is on a task, which determines the method of work (akin to a net with matrix-type structures) and with 'person culture' the individuals are central with no hierarchies (likened to a galaxy of individual stars). Handy (1993) does not claim that the descriptors can accurately define a culture; however, they can be used to gain a feel for the way an organization does things (Senior & Fleming 2006).

Reflective points

- What is the formal and informal culture within your organization and your team?
- Which of Handy's descriptors would you associate with your organization and your team (a web, temple, net or stars)?
- Does the culture of your theatre department come from the nature of anaesthesia and surgery?
- Is it determined for you or is it generated by the people who work in the department?
- Do different theatres have differing cultures or are there common cultural assumptions to all theatres?

Culture can also be explored at different levels. Schien (1997) describes three different levels, which are, from the shallowest to the deepest, artefacts level (the visible products in terms of organizational structures and processes such as environment, language, technology and style observed in values and rituals), the espoused values (the organization's strategies, goals and philosophy) and basic underlying assumptions (the unconscious, taken-for-granted beliefs, perceptions, thoughts and feelings). In order to understand a group's culture, Schien (1997) argues that its shared assumptions and how these assumptions came to be held need to be determined.

Another method to explore the culture is to examine the conflicting perceptions of culture within an organization. For instance, an NHS chief executive in the *Improvement Leaders' Guide* (Institute for Innovation and Improvement 2005) suggests that there are four organizations operating within each NHS Trust: the one that is written down, the one that most people believe exists, the one that people wished existed and, finally, the one that the organization really needs. Thus the espoused level described by Schein (1997) equates with the formal culture that is written down; the basic underlying assumptions level equates to the informal culture that staff believe exists and the artefacts level, one could argue, relates to what has worked well in the past.

Reflective points

- How would you describe the culture of your organization and your team? Are you aware of different levels?
- Is there any tension between what is written down and what you feel exists?
- Are there differences in cultural assumptions between the nurses and the operating department practitioners?
- Do these two groups have more or less in common with each other than they have with the medical staff or do people in theatres not break down into homogeneous blocks like this?

What are the unwritten rules?

The unwritten rules are one of the most powerful parts of the culture (Institute for Innovation and Improvement 2005) and, therefore, require careful consideration. From experience, it is more difficult to change culture in a mature organization than create it in a new organization. This is because the shared underlying beliefs and assumptions are implicit and unconscious (Yukl 2006). The rules are described as unwritten (Institute for Innovation and Improvement 2005) because they:

- are not often openly discussed in meetings and formal documents
- are rarely questioned or challenged

- are usually shared by most, if not all, the people who work within the team
- provide a common way for people to make sense of what is going on around them, to see situations and events in similar ways and behave accordingly
- often influence people without them necessarily realizing it
- have a powerful influence on how people behave in work.

Because people are often unaware of the unwritten rules, this makes identifying them difficult. However, as they influence most of the things we do and how we behave, we need to become politically astute by increasing our cultural awareness. By doing this we are empowered to challenge practice, ask questions and implement any required changes.

In a study by Cullen *et al.* (2000), 40 senior healthcare professionals were asked to list the unwritten rules in the NHS. Here are just a few:

- We know best
- The patient won't like it or won't want it
- Knowledge is power
- Everyone understands the jargon
- Only someone of my profession understands my problem
- Our work has no effect on other areas of the NHS
- Be honest as possible without saying anything out of line
- The more senior you are, the more you know
- Doctors know better than nurses
- I don't have to do it, someone else will
- Don't admit to mistakes
- But I've always done it that way
- Meetings = activity
- Unless there is a protocol for it, it's not happening
- Let's lie low and wait for the change to pass
- People don't change – change is hard
- I haven't got the staff or had the right training to do that
- There are no rewards for doing well
- Filling in the form makes it happen
- You have to do things cheaply
- Number of hours worked = value of outcome
- You have to work as long as the person who works the longest

- The past was much better
- Pass 'problems' up the line
- Only women do 'touchy/feely'.

Reflective points

- Do these rules sound familiar?
- Does your team have any other rules?
- Are any of the rules helpful to the promotion of a safe, innovative learning culture? If not, why not? Do any of the rules hinder innovation and change?

Does culture play a role?

A strong culture is the foundation for a strong organization (Handy 1993). Senior & Fleming (2006) support this idea and add that the greater the strength of an organization's culture the greater the degree to which it permeates all levels, and consequently the more difficult it is to influence. They suggest that one of the positive aspects of a strong culture is that it helps to avoid conflict and encourages team morale; however, a negative aspect is that a strong culture can be controlling, which can stifle innovation and change. This is particularly applicable in the health service, where cultures tend to be strong and even the smallest change requires 'jumping through hoops' and negotiating several brick walls. This is because practice tends to be based on tradition and ritual and challenging practice norms can be difficult. However, it is becoming increasingly important to justify healthcare practice and to explore the underlying evidence base. This requires all healthcare professionals to challenge the 'way we do things' and ask why. A strongly held culture is going to be more difficult to challenge and influence and so may require a different strategy to one that can be adopted in a weak culture.

Reflective points

- Is the culture of your organization strong or weak?
- What is the effect of both the organization's culture and the subculture on the management of change and team performance?

- Think about the last time a major change was introduced into your theatre. What cultural considerations were at play in promoting change and delaying change?
- What cultural assumptions drove the change through? Was it 'Lets get together and make this a success' or was it 'We have no choice but to comply' or even 'I am the boss, just do it'.

Why is understanding culture so important?

The introduction of clinical governance and the modernization agenda in the NHS recognized the importance of leadership and support to enable changes to be delivered (Department of Health 1997). The publication of *A First Class Service* (Department of Health 1998) emphasized clinical and cost-effectiveness, promotion of evidence-based practice, learning from past mistakes and involving patients and the public in the decision-making process. At this point, it was realized how much the culture and the 'way we do things' needed to change and that this would require change champions to lead and implement the reforms. The aim was to promote a culture that celebrated and encouraged success and innovation (Department of Health 1998) and this required a shift in the culture to enable and empower health-care workers to improve quality locally (Department of Health 1998). It was acknowledged that this requires visionary leaders who are motivated, self-aware, socially skilled and able to work with others (Department of Health 1999). It was also recognized that leadership is critical to the quality of care, treatment and outcomes and that poor clinical leadership leads to poor standards of care (Department of Health 2000a). *The NHS Plan* (Department of Health 2000a) also recognized the need to invest in the development of first class leaders at all levels of the NHS. The need for leadership at all levels is a theme that runs through most of the subsequent publications (Department of Health 2003, 2004a, 2005a, 2005b, 2006, 2007, 2008a, 2008b, 2008c). In addition it was recognized a culture responsive to change and sustained leadership need to be developed (Department of Health, 2004a, 2007, 2008c, 2008d). Braine (2006) argues that creating this type of culture, which embraces change and innovation, should be part of the role of every member of an organization. The aim is to create a supportive, reflective culture that encourages staff to discuss problems, report incidents and learn lessons (Braine 2006). This is a major change in working and thinking (Department of Health 2005a) that will not happen overnight and requires effort and commitment (Braine, 2006); whether these reforms are successful will depend on effective leaders (Cook 1999) at all levels of the organization. If these reforms are going to be embedded, it will require a type of leadership that inspires and motivates staff. To be successful, individual staff members need to 'buy into' the leader's vision and strategy and, most importantly, understand how this will improve the quality of patient care. It can be argued that the key to these cultural reforms is transformational leadership (Outhwaite 2003, Cook & Lethard 2004, Murphy 2005, Vincent 2006).

The role culture plays in improving patient safety is highly topical. *An Organization with a Memory* (Department of Health 2000b) states that culture can exert influence on barriers and safeguards to patient safety – for better or worse. Often the occurrence of adverse events results from poor systems, such as ineffective communication or teamwork, and often these issues themselves result from problems with leadership, culture and attitudes to patient safety (Vincent 2006). The dependency of patient safety on the culture is further highlighted by Cameron & Quinn (1999; cited by Institute for Innovation and Improvement 2005), who state that 'it is the culture . . . that influences how people think, what they see as important, how they behave and which ultimately determines the success of structural reforms'. Developing a safety culture is, therefore, a precursor to improving patient safety and reducing risk. It has also been recognized that when change does occur it takes a long time, and that the lessons from patient safety incidents have not been consistently learnt (Department of Health 2000b). It, therefore, follows that organizations need to develop a safe, open, fair blame-learning culture (National Patient Safety Agency 2004) and it is the leader's role to promote and maintain safe, high-quality patient care. An understanding of why culture is so important has evolved from a growing awareness of the issues underlying patient safety incidents/high-profile investigations and the link between reforms, change and service improvement (Institute for Innovation and Improvement 2005).

At a deeper level, it is worth considering that 'the one constant in today's healthcare environment is continuous change' (Girvin 1998:90). However, what changes all the time but stays the same? The NHS! Maybe this is because it is acknowledged that implementing change is important but it is difficult (Yukl 2006). The first step to improvement is to convince people to leave the safety of their 'home area' (Bridges 2003; cited by Institute for Innovation and Improvement 2005) and, therefore, the challenge is to inspire staff with your vision so they are convinced the change will be mutually beneficial. The reason why so many change projects fail is neglect of the human dimensions of change (Institute for Innovation and Improvement 2005). This means failure to involve staff, communicate the vision effectively and justify the reasons why change should occur plus failure to listen to staff, act on their ideas and recognize their emotions and feelings, particularly fear. So the next step after initiating a change project is to involve staff so they are committed to coming up with the solutions to the problem (Lewin 1951; cited by Yakl 2006), and in this way their involvement will act as a catalyst for change (Covey 1992).

At a more visible level, culture affects practices and procedures (Sullivan & Decker 2005) both within the organization and within the team. Consider the following. Are patients/carers empowered to take responsibility for their care? Are research and audit encouraged? How much emphasis is placed on, and time devoted to, staff development? How are policies and guidelines enforced and are they adhered to? How is the uniform policy enforced? Are staff members permitted to leave theatre in 'greens'? Do the same rules apply to all

groups in this policy or only some groups? How accurate is documentation? How long is lunch time? Are staff members encouraged to be involved in the decision-making and problem-solving process? Are staff members permitted to challenge decisions? For example, it is unlikely that there is a written policy about whether junior staff members are permitted to question decisions made by senior staff or managers but most staff will know if it is acceptable or frowned upon. Do all staff speak up at meetings or are meetings dominated by one professional group?

Culture also has an impact on team and individual performance, which, in turn, impacts on quality, performance, motivation and job satisfaction. For instance, a study was undertaken by Davies *et al.* (2007) to explore the relationship between senior management, team culture and organizational performance in 197 English NHS Acute Trusts. They used a culture-rating instrument (competing values framework) to assess senior management team culture and they found a direct relationship between culture and performance. Furthermore, an article in the *Nursing Times* (Smy, 2007) highlights the need to listen and act on nurses' views; the respondents to the questionnaire singled out the importance of having a strong voice at every level of the organization. A consistent theme was a need for respect and for their work to be valued. Having a voice and being valued was 'powerfully motivating' as this was felt to raise standards and improve job satisfaction (Smy 2007:16). Further research has shown the importance of culture in contributing towards high-quality patient care (Institute for Innovation and Improvement 2005). For example, in a study of over 5000 patients in intensive care, significant differences in death rates between hospitals were found despite similar staffing levels, funding and populations. These differences appeared to be related to the quality of interaction and communication between healthcare professionals (Knaus 1986; cited by Institute for Innovation and Improvement 2005).

An awareness of culture will, therefore, facilitate influencing a team's performance, implementing change effectively and improving staff motivation. In addition, involving staff in the decision-making process and demonstrating action following such consultation will not only improve quality and patient safety but will also have a positive impact on staff morale and, again, motivation. This encourages the team to 'go the extra mile' and have real pride in their work. In this way, the attitudes and vision of a leader can have a positive impact on the culture of the organization (Faugier & Woolnough 2002).

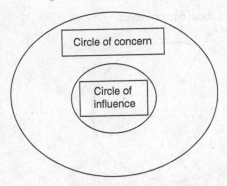

Figure 12.1 Circles of concern and influence.

Reflective points

- How will your cultural awareness inform the way you behave and inspire your team and inform the way you implement change?
- How does culture impact on the practices and procedures in your work place?
- Are there any aspects to 'theatre culture' you think ought to be challenged? What about 'gallows humour'? Is this a collective coping mechanism or is it something you regard as unprofessional?
- Can the notion of 'professional' be explained in anything other than a cultural way?

Culture and change

It is evident that culture has a dominant influence on the whole organization (Senior & Fleming 2006) and, therefore, to implement change successfully a leader must be politically aware and be able to positively influence the culture. Major change usually requires a change in the culture (Yukl 2006) and permanent change will only happen by first changing people's attitudes and values (Senior & Fleming 2006). So how is change implemented successfully in the NHS and how can an individual know what is within their control to change? A good starting point may be to consider what is within their sphere of influence, in other words to be aware of what can and what cannot be changed. A useful tool to illustrate this is Covey's (1992) circles of concern/influence (Fig. 12.1). The tool can be utilized as a self-awareness exercise to

determine a personal degree of proactivity and thus empower for implementing change. Covey (1992) argues that everyone has a wide range of concerns; however, some of these concerns are ones over which they have no real control and others are amenable to change.

Reflective points

- Using Fig. 12.1, draw a circle of concern and add all your concerns about the culture of your organization and team. Consider the attitudes and values of both the organization and your team. Now consider the concerns that you can do something about and circumscribe them within a smaller circle of influence (Fig. 12.2).
- Which of the issues (within your circle of concern) are within your power to influence?

Covey (1989:82) argues that by determining which of these two circles is the focus of most of our time and energy we can discover much about the 'degree of our proactivity'. Proactive leaders focus their efforts in their circle of influence, that is, they are aware of what they can do something about and concentrate on these areas. As their energy and influence is positive, it causes their circle of influence to enlarge and their confidence to grow. However reactive leaders focus on their circle of concern, that is the things that they have no control over. As this energy is very negative, they fail to do something positive where they have the power to do so and their circle of influence shrinks (Covey 1989).

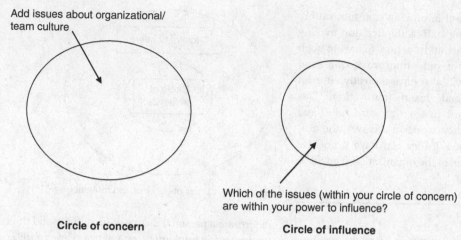

Add issues about organizational/
team culture

Which of the issues (within your circle of concern)
are within your power to influence?

Circle of concern   **Circle of influence**

Figure 12.2 Using circles of concern and influence.

Furthermore, Covey (1989:84) argues that if we continue to work in our circle of concern 'we empower the things within it to control us'. By working within our sphere of influence, we are 'consciously' in control; we have the power to choose our responses and we are empowered to implement change, problem solve and be creative. This is opposed to being a 'victim', where control is lost and change is forced upon you or having a defeatist attitude of 'anything I do will make no difference'.

> **Reflective points**
>
> • What are the issues within your circle of concern that you can influence?
> • Where and how will you now direct your energy?

How is culture related to leadership?

Culture is not stable; it is something that develops and changes over time (Palmer 2001) and it can be strongly influenced by the leadership styles of key personnel. This means that an individual can make a difference. In fact, if an individual can understand the environment, he or she can then plan how to respond to it (Yukl 2006).

Cultures are moulded by 'events of the past, the climate of the present, by the technology ... by [organization's] aims and the kind of people that work within them' (Handy 1993:180). In order for leaders to be effective, they need to be aware of the culture within their organization and team otherwise the culture will manage them (Schein 1997). Successful leaders are also proactive, taking the lead, and this requires taking ownership of the challenges that occur and the responsibility for finding solutions. This, in turn, requires leaders to build effective teams and to empower their staff to implement the team's vision and philosophy of care. It is important at this point to reflect on what was discussed above about spheres of influence (Covey 1989) to ensure that energy is focused on what can be changed. If a manager enlarges his or her sphere of influence, this empowers both manager and the team and has a positive impact on their circle of concern.

How can you determine the culture within an organization?

A starting point to explore how an organization and team would like their culture to develop is

Table 12.1 Indications of the type of culture at a macro- and microlevel

Macro indication (organization level)	Micro indications (team level)
Themes from complaints and incidents	Effective, high-performing teams
Type of safety culture: blame, fair blame, no blame	Effective communication
Quality indicators (annual health check, clinical governance assessments)	Multiprofessional collaboration
Compliance with risk management standards	Multidisciplinary team working
Internal/external audit	Staff satisfaction
Patient/user feedback	Conflict management
Staff recruitment and retention, 'staff exit' questionnaires	Quality of care
Effective two-way communication	Staff morale
Staff involved in decision-making process	Staff ownership and responsibility
Evidence of lessons learnt from incidents and complaints	Patient empowerment
Stakeholder feedback	Staff involved in decision making
Publicity	Problem solving with evidence of action

to evaluate their philosophies of care. When was the philosophy written? Is it current? Who wrote the philosophy and for what purpose? Were all staff groups involved? Does it reflect your goals, vision and aspirations? Are members of staff aware of the philosophy? Does it reflect their views? Does it meet the needs of patients, carers and staff? It is then important to consider if the team's philosophy reflects that of the organization. This could be demonstrated if the team member's personal objectives are aligned with the ward/departments objectives and these, in turn, are linked to those of the organization. Once an understanding of the rationale underpinning the philosophy is gained, consider if a new shared philosophy needs to be written by the multidisciplinary team.

To help in thinking about and determining the culture of a particular team, consider the following five questions, which are based on the *Improvement Leaders Guide* (Institute for Innovation and Improvement 2005):

Decision-making. Who is involved? Do these people represent the multidisciplinary team? Are both senior and junior staff involved?

Communication. Do you use a range of communication channels, both formal and informal?

Teamwork. Does the team consist of a group of individuals or an effective team with a common purpose and shared vision?

Handling conflict. Are issues discussed openly and constructively?

Change and innovation. Does the team have a proactive approach to change, continuously looking for new ways of working? Does the team brainstorm ideas and look for creative solutions to problems?

This analysis will give a 'feel' for the culture and an understanding of the way staff think, work and how situations are dealt with within the team. The issues discussed above could be considered if an understanding of the culture at a deeper level is needed:

- the formal and informal cultures (Palmer 2001)
- what type of culture is operating (Handy 1993)
- what are the values and behaviours
- what are the unwritten rules (Cullen *et al.* 2000).

This information can then be linked to the issues discussed subsequently:

- the organization's safety culture
- the macro- and microlevel indicators (Table 12.1)
- the recruitment preferences for key leadership positions (Sullivan & Decker 2005).

It is difficult to put the indicators in Table 12.1 into just one of the columns as it is clear that there is a lot

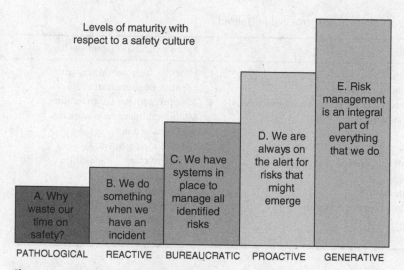

Levels of maturity with respect to a safety culture

A. Why waste our time on safety?

B. We do something when we have an incident

C. We have systems in place to manage all identified risks

D. We are always on the alert for risks that might emerge

E. Risk management is an integral part of everything that we do

PATHOLOGICAL   REACTIVE   BUREAUCRATIC   PROACTIVE   GENERATIVE

Figure 12.3 The Manchester Patient Safety Framework tool.

of overlap between the micro- and macrolevel indicators, but the indicators should provide a catalyst for reflection and will allow consideration as to whether there are any other applicable indicators.

Another method of measuring the organization's culture, which is both highly topical and applicable to the NHS, is to determine the safety culture. The reason that this is so important is that patient safety is partly determined by the attitudes and values of staff (Vincent 2006). For example, measuring the safety culture will provide a good indication of the type and maturity of the culture embedded within the organization. Determining the safety culture not only provides a focus as to where challenges lie but also provides an insight into whether the organization is reactive or proactive. This affects, for example, how conflict is managed, how change is received, whether the culture is open or closed and if lessons are learnt and, in turn, it will influence communication and teamwork. An awareness of the safety culture will also help to determine where resistance to change is likely because of incompatibility between strategy and culture (Senior & Fleming 2006). This, in turn, provides an opportunity to consider an approach and helps in making an informed decision on how to manage the situation. For example, the culture could be a

restraining or driving force (Lewin 1951; cited by Yukl 2006); so does the culture need to be changed to fit the project (or whatever change is intended) or the project changed to fit the culture?

To help in understanding the safety culture within healthcare, the National Patient Safety Agency (NPSA) has collaborated with Manchester University to develop a safety culture tool. The NPSA is a Special Health Authority with responsibility for improving patient safety in organizations providing NHS-funded care and the tool is based on *The 7 Steps to Patient Safety* (Department of Health 2004b). The tool for reflecting on the safety culture is concerned with the first one of the seven steps, building a safety culture. Reflection on the safety culture provides an insightful evaluation of the maturity of the culture within the organization and also an indication of its strengths and weaknesses. The NPSA have defined a safety culture as:

- where staff have a constant and active awareness of the potential for things to go wrong
- open and fair and one that encourages people to speak up about mistakes.

The Manchester Patient Safety Framework tool (Fig. 12.3; National Patient Safety Agency 2004). was initially used in primary care but there is now a version specifically for mental health, and for

Acute

Aspect of patient safety culture	A	B	C	D	E
1. Commitment to overall continuous improvement					
2. Priority given to safety					
3. System errors and individual responsibility					
4. Recording incidents and best practice					
5. Evaluating incidents and best practice					
6. Learning and effecting change					
7. Communication about safety issues					
8. Personnel management and safety issues					
9. Staff education and training					
10. Team working					

Figure 12.4 Format for completion of the Manchester Patient Safety Framework tool; items A–E are defined in Figure 12.3.

acute and ambulance trusts. Five different types of organization are defined in terms of how they process information: pathological, reactive, bureaucratic, proactive and generative.

The tool is completed following consideration of different aspects of the safety culture and can be completed in terms of a specific organization or team (Fig. 12.4). This enables culture to be explored from examination of the philosophy of both the organization and the team and the behaviour of the teams. The evidence can be gathered from the micro- and macrolevel indicators and specific evaluation of the safety culture.

Reflective points

• What is the culture within your organization and team?
• What actions do you need to take to move your team to the next level of the safety culture? Consider Covey's (1992) circles of concern/influence in order to determine your proactive response.
• Do you believe that these models of organization have any bearing on your theatre? Or are 'one size fits all' models of no use in the very particular circumstances of a busy operating theatre?

Organizational development continuum

The influence of a leader on the culture is directly related to the development stage of the organization (Yukl 2006). So a starting point is to consider the stage of development and whether the culture is mature or is still evolving. Handy (1993) argues that organizations gradually change their dominant culture and although most start as power cultures, the culture changes through growth and maturity (e.g. when the organization's success is no longer dependent on the chief executive). If power is delegated and decision making shared, then a role culture may develop (Handy 1993). The next change comes when the organization realizes greater flexibility is required in order to compete and stay ahead of the competition, for example through the use of technology. The key then is to find the appropriate cultural diversity (Handy 1993); in other words, organizations need to adapt to change continually and adopt the most appropriate culture. For example, the accident and emergency department (power culture: the management of crisis) should be organized in a different way to the outpatient department (role culture: routine procedures, clinical guidelines, policy). However, there will be times when a different approach is required: consider the effect of restructuring, new staff, new management or new vision/purpose.

Attention must also be paid to the trust–control relationship, which according to Handy (1993) needs to be complementary. If control is high, trust is low. An increase in trust is only achieved and, therefore, only effective, if a reduction in control occurs in tandem (Handy 1993). Furthermore, in a low-trust culture, it is difficult to empower staff and thus embed win–win agreements or promote self-supervision and self-evaluation (Covey 1992).

Once the nature of the culture is understood, consideration can be given to its level of maturity and the trust–control relationship. This will inform strategies for how to influence it.

Reflective points

- Where is your organization on the development continuum?
- Do you have a high or low degree of trust and control?
- How does your organization's development relate to the level of safety maturity (the NPSA model)?

The leadership role

Effective leadership is recognized as being critical to the modernization of the NHS and this, together with teamwork, effective communication, ownership and systems awareness, forms the foundation of clinical governance (Braine 2006). An awareness of the organizational culture and how it works is essential in order to appreciate the complexities and help in identifying where a manager fits in and what leadership role they play. The role of the manager in the development of highly performing empowered teams cannot be underestimated. Teamwork lies at the heart of any cultural shift (Cullen *et al.* 2000) and the first steps are a shared philosophy, vision and mutually agreed values, behaviours and standards of care. The team manager needs to sell his or her vision of a better future in order to move people out of

their comfort zone and into sharing these aspirations. At the same time, the manager needs to be able justify the hardships and sacrifices the change will bring (Yukl 2006). Once there is commitment from the staff, the next step is to create a climate that allows teams to reflect, be creative and problem solve in a supportive environment. This environment needs to be open and questioning (Cullen *et al.* 2000).

The key to cultural change is empowerment of staff so that the organization becomes a learning organization. When clinical leaders are empowered they can influence the broader culture of an organization (Smith & Edmonstone 2001). What is meant by empowerment? Simply put, empowerment means 'letting go so others can get going' (Blanchard 1994:110). This means leaders need to 'skill up' staff, clearly communicate their vision and involve staff in the decision-making process so staff have a vested interest in providing solutions to the daily problems. Leaders who can achieve this have the ability to inspire staff to challenge ritualistic practice and to empower staff to think of creative, 'third option' solutions. According to Covey (1992), an empowered organization is one in which individuals have the knowledge, skill, desire and opportunity to succeed personally in a way that leads to collective success. This can only happen if power and responsibility are delegated and the culture supports change, creativity, innovation and fair blame. In other words, the organization becomes a learning organization. Braine (2006) argues that this requires clinical governance to be embedded into everyday practice, the culture needs to support critical inquiry and lifelong learning; members of staff need to embrace accountability and responsibility, and the organization needs to be reflective so that failures are openly discussed and lessons are learnt. Furthermore, Hardacre (2001) describes a learning organization as one that is continuously ready for change, evolution and transformation, and that this requires a safe, supportive environment built on a continuous cycle of learning and improvement.

In order to nurture empowerment in organizations there are six conditions that need to be in place (Covey 1992):

1. *win–win agreements*: to motivate staff to align organizational goals with personal objectives
2. *self-supervision*: staff should supervise themselves in terms of their objectives (in the win–win agreement)
3. *accountability*: staff are performance managed against their agreed objectives via self-evaluation
4. *helpful structures and systems*: to support self-directing, self-controlling individuals to fulfil their win–win agreement (e.g. job design, information, communication, constructive feedback about performance, training and development)
5. *skills awareness*: what a person can do (e.g. communication, problem solving, planning) related to the *Knowledge and Skills Framework* (KSF)
6. *character awareness*: what a person is (e.g. values, maturity, action).

The last two, skills and character, are the competencies required to establish and maintain the other four; that is, the foundations required to establish trusting relationships, win–win agreements, self-supervision and self-evaluation. According to Covey (1992), the six conditions are so interdependent that if any one of them is out of balance it will affect the other five, so a leader's role is to embed the six conditions and then monitor closely.

The leader's role is, therefore, to embed quality and patient safety into routine practice, become a 'change champion', empower the team and create a learning climate.

Reflective point

- How will you nurture empowerment within your team and organization?

How can culture be influenced?

The place to start is personally, and this is probably the most important step: self-reflection. However, understanding yourself is not easy (Jooste 2004); it takes time and a great deal of soul searching. So a manager may need to reflect on and explore his or her own values and beliefs initially and then strive to develop self-awareness (Outhwaite 2003) of strengths, weaknesses and areas for personal development. It is important that self-leadership comes before leading others, and this means setting personal aims and objectives as well as high standards of care and communication (Adair 2006).

Reflection does not stop with the person. It is also important to consider behaviour and attitude towards the team and the type of team culture that the manager is aspiring to develop. Is there any tension between personal philosophy (principles, the type of leader you are aspiring to become and the type of culture you would like to develop) and behaviour? It is recognized that leaders need to develop their own team (Outhwaite 2003, Adair, 2006); however, it is also worth remembering that a manager is only as good as the team he or she leads. The manager is the team's role model and the way managers act and behave, and what they say and how they say it, has a profound effect on their team. The aim is to empower others to act and fulfil their potential (Adair 2006) through leading by example, support and guidance. A critical factor in determining the success of highly performing teams is principle-centred leadership (Hardacre 2001). Principle-centred leadership is based on *The 7 Habits of Highly Effective People* (Covey 1989) and because it focuses on fundamental principles and processes, cultural transformations often occur (Covey 1992). The seven habits are as follows.

1. Be proactive: based on self-awareness. Responses to external stimuli are a value-based choices or responses; take the initiative (think about expanding your circle of influence).
2. Begin with the end in mind: based on clear thinking. Start with a clear understanding of what you want to achieve and this will inform the direction and action you take: your vision (what can you do within your circle of influence).
3. Put first things first: based on willpower. Time management ensures that you are in control and are dealing with prevention rather than crisis.

4. Think win–win: based on seeking agreement. It is better to find solutions that are mutually beneficial and mutually satisfying; this is the third alternative (not your way or my way but a better, higher way).

5. Seek first to understand, then to be understood: based on courage balanced with consideration. Use empathic listening to enable the problem to be understood first; this is the key to effective interpersonal communication.

6. Synergise: based on creativity. The whole is greater than the sum of the parts so value differences, build on strengths, compensate for weaknesses (teamwork), which leads to a synergistic third alternative where solutions are better than either side initially proposed.

7. Sharpen the saw: based on continuous improvement and preserving and enhancing your greatest asset (you). This ensures a healthy, balanced life, with physical, spiritual, mental and social/emotional self-renewal.

So the seven habits teach us to lead by example, reflect on and renew our skills, treat others as we would expect to be treated ourselves and value teamwork. In addition, when a manager is empowered from within (Covey 1992), he or she is both governed and grounded by these core principles. This allows the manager to maintain judgement in times of crisis and provides insight and balance (e.g. with ethical dilemmas), thus providing a guiding light and a strong frame of reference. The habits encourage leadership through modelling behaviour and this has a pivotal influence on moving staff in the right direction and influencing culture. The habits are actions that a manager should strive to develop over time and with experience, interpreting them at new higher levels as his or her leadership skills mature.

To summarize, in order for an individual to grow and develop these habits, it is first important to be self-aware and then through experience and reflection to learn if personal principles are enacted.

An eight-step reflective model for cultural awareness

This section summarizes what has been discussed in this chapter and proposes an 'eight-step reflective model' that can be utilized to raise cultural awareness and thus determine how you can influence the culture. The model is based on a figure of eight (Fig. 12.5). The aim of the model is to allow places to stop and think, thus providing opportunities to choose and plan responses. For each step, additional questions have been proposed to guide understanding (Fig. 12.5).

Step 1 is reflection to aid self-awareness (as discussed above).

Steps 2–4 are exploration and evidence gathering. These three steps involve exploring the formal/informal culture and unwritten rules in order to gain a deeper understanding of the organization. What are the shared values of the organization and the team? Identify as many behaviours as possible and compare these with the stated values and behaviours. Search for the unwritten rules and consider how they came about and why they persist.

Step 5 is critical analysis. Here any tensions between what is written and the realities of practice in terms of the informal, formal, team and organizational culture are considered. Following this analysis, how can the organization and team be described in terms of Handy's (1993) descriptors, the micro- and macrolevel indicators, with respect to safety maturity and where the organization sits on the development continuum. This step may result in return back around the top circle (of the figure of eight figure) again, as following analysis it may be determined that further reflection is required and this, in turn, may require further information. Progress to the lower circle only occurs once you are confident you have sufficient insight.

Step 6 is reflection. Here is the point at which consideration is given as to what can and cannot be influenced in terms of your sphere of influence.

Step 7 is action. Action is taken in light of your principles and values, vision and aspirations (aims

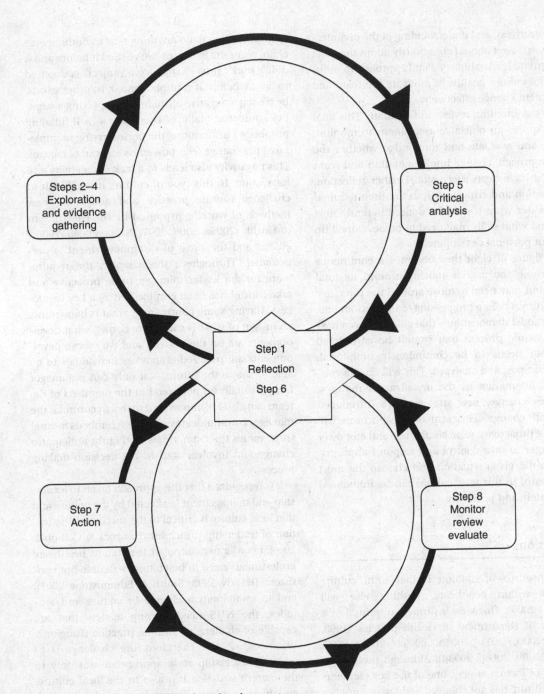

Figure 12.5 The eight-step model for cultural awareness.

and objectives), and understanding of the organization. A manager should consciously adopt the most appropriate leadership style and approach to influence the culture positively, motivate the team and implement change effectively.

Step 8 is monitor, review and evaluate. This final step requires an objective assessment to monitor, review and evaluate and thus judge whether the style/approach, change implementation and team building have been successful. Further reflection, information and critical analysis are then required to consider what should be done differently next time and what skills may need to be developed (in terms of personal development).

The figure of eight thus becomes a continuous loop where the user is moving around its total length but may need to move around the top circle several times before progressing to the bottom one.

The model demonstrates that cultural awareness is a dynamic process that cannot be considered once but needs to be continuously monitored, reflected upon and analysed. This will enable continuous adaptation as the organization matures, priorities change, new strategies are introduced and staff change. This structured approach will promote proactivity, raise confidence and empower a manager to take control and respond appropriately to the given situation and choose the most direct path. In this way, culture can be influenced deliberately and positively.

Conclusions

The consensus of opinion is that until culture changes within healthcare, nothing else will (Vincent 2006). This view is further supported by a plethora of Department of Health policies (1998, 1999, 2000b, 2003, 2004b, 2005a, 2006, 2007, 2008a, 2008b, 2008c, 2008d). Although there are a number of factors at play, one of the key elements in why culture has not changed and lessons are not learnt (Department of Health 2000b) is a feeling of futility: that a person is a slave to the culture and not master of it. This has led to attitudes of it being

pointless trying to do anything new as nothing ever changes for the better, or 'we've tried it before and it didn't work'; thus change (or a project) is doomed to failure before it is implemented. In other words, by having a negative attitude and expecting a negative outcome, failure becomes a self-fulfilling prophecy. Furthermore, the person trying to implement the change feels powerless and out of control. This negativity also leads to a lack of creativity and innovation. In this type of culture, it is difficult to challenge routine practice and adopt the new methods of working espoused by the Department of Health (2005a, 2006, 2007, 2008a, 2008b, 2008c, 2008d) and the cycle of disempowerment is perpetuated. Throughout this chapter, the requirement for the leader/manager to be proactive and take control has been emphasized as a key to success. Having some control over what is happening, an insight of what is round the corner, what developments are on the horizon and why these developments are required empowers individuals to be able to shape the future. Not only can a manager feel personally empowered but the members of the team can also be empowered to feel in control if the manager communicates effectively, embeds mutual trust, values the team, treats staff fairly, anticipates change and involves staff in the decision-making process.

It is recognized that the approach taken to leadership and management is affected by the culture and that local culture is critical to the successful application of leadership principles (Hancock & Campbell 2006). In order to manipulate the culture, healthcare professionals need to be culturally flexible but consistent (Handy 1993, Smith & Edmonstone 2001), and to implement a change in culture and attitudes, the NHS needs strong leaders that are capable of challenging routine practice (Faugier & Woolnough 2002). Therefore, the challenge is to adopt a leadership style appropriate not only to the current situation but also to the local culture, and in my opinion principle-centred leadership provides the solution. Principle-centred leaders empower staff, challenge current mindsets, take risks, innovate, have a common vision, anticipate change and take ownership and responsibility (Cullen *et al.* 2000). To create a culture that celebrates and encourages success and innovation and that acknowledges and learns from past mistakes (Department of Health 1998) requires a culture that is patient-centred, encourages improvement and innovation, recognizes the value of learning, is based on honesty and trust and promotes effective teamworking and two-way communication (Institute for Innovation and Improvement 2005). This supportive climate is demonstrated by day-to-day leadership behaviour, by setting an example (Larson & Lafasto 1989). Thus effective leadership not only empowers staff but also creates a culture that is open to change and innovation (Braine 2006). Consequently, cultural manipulation requires transformational principle-centred leadership: that is, leaders who challenge the way things are done and what the organization does and who lead change through engagement and collaboration.

In summary, it is within the control of a manager to influence culture and empower the team. A manager does have the power to bring about change (Jooste 2004) and one person can be a change catalyst, a transformer in an organization (Covey 1992). The initial step is self-belief – to believe you can make a difference – if you do not believe it, how will you inspire others? It is important, however, for a manager to think very carefully about why the culture needs influencing or the change implemented and how it is proposed to do that. This is so that, first, there is a clear vision that staff can commit to and, second, the manager is focused and sets achievable outcomes that are linked to improvements in patient care. Changing the cultural paradigm is not easy nor will it happen overnight but it can be done. It requires sustained effort based on transformational principle-centred leadership, not quick-fix solutions. Providing the right culture allows the right attitudes and behaviours to flourish (Vincent 2006) and it is on these foundations that the leaders of tomorrow will grow. This fertile culture is a reward worth striving for. The journey begins with self-reflection and the path takes an endless loop (or figure of eight) of continuous reflection, critical analysis, anticipation of change and finally adaptation to change.

REFERENCES

Adair, J. (2006). *Not Bosses but Leaders*, 3rd edn. London: Kogan Page.

Blanchard, K. (1994). *The One Minute Manager*. London: Harper Collins.

Braine, M. (2006). Clinical governance: applying theory to practice. *Nursing Standard*, **20**, 56–65.

Cook, M. J. (1999). Improving care requires leadership in nursing. *Nurse Education Today*, **19**, 306–312.

Cook, M. J. & Lethard, H. (2004). Learning for clinical leadership. *Journal of Nursing Management*, **12**, 436–444.

Cullen, R., Nicholas, S. & Halligan, A. (2000). Reviewing a service: discovering the unwritten rules. *British Journal of Clinical Governance*, **5**, 233–239.

Covey, S. (1989). *The 7 Habits of Highly Effective People*. London: Simon and Schuster.

Covey, S. (1992). *Principle-Centred Leadership*. London: Simon and Schuster.

Davies, H., Mannion, R., Jacobs, R., Power, A. & Marshall, M. (2007). Is there an association between senior management team culture and hospital performance? *Medical Care Research and Review*, **64**, 46–65.

Department of Health (1997). *The New NHS Modern, Dependable*. London: The Stationery Office.

Department of Health (1998). *A First Class Service*. London: The Stationery Office.

Department of Health (1999). *Making a Difference: Strengthening the Nursing, Midwifery and Health Visiting Contribution to Health and Healthcare*. London: The Stationery Office.

Department of Health (2000a). *The NHS Plan: A Plan for Investment, a Plan for Reform*. London: The Stationery Office.

Department of Health (2000b). *An Organisation with a Memory*. London: The Stationery Office.

Department of Health (2003). *Raising Standards: Improving Performance in the NHS*. London: The Stationery Office.

Department of Health (2004a). *The NHS Improvement Plan: Putting People at the Heart of Public Services*. London: The Stationery Office.

Department of Health (2004b). *The 7 Steps to Patient Safety: An Overview Guide for NHS Staff*. London: The Stationery Office.

Department of Health (2005a). *Creating a Patient-led NHS: Delivering the NHS Improvement Plan*. London: The Stationery Office.

Department of Health (2005a). *Independence, Wellbeing and Choice: Our Vision for the Future of Social Care for Adults in England*. London: The Stationery Office.

Department of Health (2006). *Our Health, Our Care, Our Say*. London: The Stationery Office.

Department of Health (2007). *Our NHS, Our Future: NHS Next Stage Review. Interim Report*. London: The Stationery Office.

Department of Health (2008a). *High Quality Care for All. NHS Next Stage Review Final Report*. London: The Stationery Office.

Department of Health (2008a). *A High Quality Workforce: NHS Next Stage Review*. London: The Stationery Office.

Department of Health (2008c). *Our NHS, Our Future*. London: The Stationery Office.

Department of Health (2008d). *Changing for the Better: Guidance when Undertaking Major Changes to NHS Services*. London: The Stationery Office.

Faugier, J. & Woolnough, H. (2002). Valuing 'voices from below'. *Journal of Nursing Management*, **10**, 315–320.

Girvin, J. (1998). *Leadership in Nursing*. Basingstoke, UK: McMillan.

Hancock, H. & Campbell, S. (2006). Impact of the Leading and Empowered Organisation Programme. *Nursing Standard*, **20**, 41–48.

Handy, C. (1993). *Understanding Organisations*, 4th edn. London: Penguin.

Hardacre, J. (2001). *Health Service Journal Management Academy: Leadership at Every Level*. London: Emap Public Sector Management.

Institute for Innovation and Improvement (2005). *Improvement Leaders Guide*. Warwick: Institute for Innovation and Improvement; www.institute.nhs.uk (accessed 20 April 2009).

Jooste, K. (2004). Leadership:a new perspective. *Journal of Nursing Management*, **12**, 217–223.

Larson, C. & Lafasto, F. (1989). *Teamwork: What Must Go Right, What Can Go Wrong*. London: Sage.

Murphy, L. (2005). Transformational leadership: a cascading chain reaction. *Journal of Nursing Management*, **13**, 128–136.

National Patient Safety Agency (2004). *Delivering safer health care*. London: National Patient Safety Agency; www.npsa.nhs.uk (accessed 20 April 2009).

Outhwaite, S. (2003). The importance of leadership in the development of an integrated team. *Journal of Nursing Management*, **11**, 371–376.

Palmer, S. (2001). *People and Self Management*. Oxford: Butterworth-Heinemann.

Schein, E. (1997). *Organisational Culture and Leadership*, 2nd edn. San Francisco, CA: Jossey-Bass.

Senior, B. & Fleming, J. (2006). *Organisational Change*, 3rd edn. London: Pearson Education.

Smith, S. & Edmonstone, J. (2001). Learning to lead. *Nursing Management*, **8**, 10–13.

Smy, J. (2007). The value of being a good employer of nurses. *Nursing Times*, **103**, 38–42.

Sullivan, E. & Decker, P. (2005). *Effective Leadership and Management in Nursing*. Upper Saddle River, NJ: Pearson Prentice Hall.

Vincent, C. (2006). *Patient Safety*. Elsevier: Churchill Livingstone.

Yukl, G. (2006). *Leadership in Organisations*, 6th edn. Upper Saddle River, NJ: Pearson Prentice Hall.

13

Development matters in the NHS; *including a perioperative approach to the KSF*

Lorraine Thomas

Key Learning points

- A discussion of the relationship between national health service development and education
- Current influences on and key aspects of professional development
- Fundamental factors in implementation of the Knowledge and Skills Framework
- A practical approach to PDP evidence collection and recording for perioperative practitioners

Development matters in the NHS

The cumulative effect of several significant Department of Health (DH) initiatives has arguably contributed to the current emphasis on performance development within the National Health Service (NHS). Consideration of the literature suggests that policy appears to be driven by two key and connected aspects of reform: modernization of services including, the efficiency and effectiveness of those services; and continuing development of health care professionals. Directives including the introduction of the National Patient Safety Agency – Building a safer NHS for Patients (DH 2001), Creating a Patient-led NHS (DH 2005a) and the development of Foundation Trusts (DH 2005c) are instrumental to the modernization agenda and strive to ensure a safe approach to care that is not only patient focused but patient led. Initiatives supporting continuing professional development, including Modernizing Medical Careers (DH 2004a),

Modernizing Nursing Careers (DH 2006c), and the regulation of Health Professionals in the twenty-first century (Secretary of State 2007) could be considered the vehicles by which service developments may be achieved. The DH (2004c) would appear to support this view, introducing the aim of Agenda for Change (AfC) Knowledge and Skills Framework (KSF) as 'the development of services so that they better meet the needs of service users and the public through investing in the development of all members of staff' (DH 2004c, p. 3). This perspective places service delivery as a main focus of health care services with education and staff development in a secondary or supporting role. This approach undoubtedly describes at least one function of education, as it could be argued that any health service improvement necessitates some degree of education to facilitate its implementation and the wider the application of the initiative the more standardized and robust the educational programmes have the potential to be. A number of NHS-wide initiatives demonstrate a direct link between education and service improvement, suggesting education to be pivotal in improving structures and systems of care. The current emphasis on developing existing roles and responsibilities is evident and wide reaching. The DH document Modernizing Medical Careers (DH 2004a) aims to reform post-graduate medical education and defines the driver for change as 'the need for better care systems for patients' (DH 2004a, p. 1). A similar

Core Topics in Operating Department Practice: Leadership and Management, ed. Brian Smith, Paul Rawling, Paul Wicker and Chris Jones. Published by Cambridge University Press. © Cambridge University Press 2010.

approach to reform is taken with Modernizing Nursing Careers (DH 2006c). This document refers to the 'profound changes taking place in the structure of health care delivery' and seeks to support nurses in 'flexible, diverse and rewarding careers' (DH 2006c p. 3). The National Practitioner Programme aims to support role development with the Anaesthesia Practitioner (DH 2005b), Surgical Care Practitioner (DH 2006a) and Advanced Scrub Practitioner (Perioperative Care Collaborative 2007) amongst those initiatives designed to improve perioperative service development. The portfolio of programmes aims to support post-graduate and post-registration career pathways and new ways of working, including assisting non-medical professionals to perform what are traditionally considered medical roles.

The DH modernization agenda is additionally supported by professional regulatory organizations notably the General Medical Council (GMC) (2006), Nursing and Midwifery Council (NMC) (2008b, 2006) and Health Professions Council (HPC) (2008a, 2008c) (HPC 2008b), who similarly advocate the influence of continuing professional development in achieving improvements in health care provision.

Accepting that education plays a significant role in supporting service improvements, a surface approach might be to perceive professional development as an essential tool in implementing best practice and therefore a useful and necessary accompaniment to service development. This approach is arguably supported by the fact that the concept of health care service delivery is generally defined in a way that is almost synonymous with the concept of patient care. Certainly, the collective approach of the health professions (NMC 2008a), (HPC 2008a) (GMC 2006) is to uphold the provision of safe and effective patient care as the primary guiding principle of professional practice and that remains beyond question. Arguably, however, the term service delivery can only be defined as synonymous with patient care when it represents a quality service with a focus on individual needs. Such a model remains the primary aim of the modernization agenda and a

reality towards which the NHS continues to strive. This is evident from the requirement for the introduction of the National Patient Safety Agency, the implementation of the DH initiative an organization with a memory (DH 2001), the launch of Valuing People (DH 2009) and the recent and significant initiative Safe Surgery Saves Lives (World Health Organization) (WHO) (2008). All of these documents highlight the need for improvement in health care delivery systems and in some cases an urgent need (WHO 2008). An environment where much is still to be achieved in terms of quality health care services and staff development presents a considerable challenge for education and educators and it would seem that modernization initiatives are both significant in number and increasing, with each apparently requiring some level of educational response. Whilst this environment continues, education services could be considered a supporting, but not a secondary, service as it provides an essential resource in achieving NHS goals. Accepting adequate resources, it is more than probable that education in the form of instruction or imparting and dissemination of knowledge can achieve the implementation and embedding of quality systems, standardization of best practice and, to some degree, new ways of working. If, however, education is to be utilized to its optimum benefit, then the NHS has the opportunity to harness the role of education as the initiator of the health care innovations including the patient involvement programmes it is striving to achieve.

It could be argued that the value of a resource is most apparent in its absence. The question of whether, in the absence of health education, an effective health service would exist could provoke an interesting hypothesis and an intriguing line of enquiry. It could, of course, prove problematic to test such a hypothesis and in view of the current reliance on education services, it may be more appropriate to acknowledge that the validity of some phenomena can be accepted without being subject to the rigour of scientific method (Pell and Smith 2003).

An alternative approach may be to contemplate health care practice from a relatively recent, historic perspective (Ellis 2009; Nightingale 2006) and consider the contribution of education to the development of quality health services. Arguably, this demonstrates that education in its widest sense, i.e. including experiential learning, reflection and research serves not only as a vehicle to implement service developments, but is in some instances the catalyst for, or instigator of, fundamental and reformative service developments. Consideration of the two services from this perspective raises perceptions of education from a position of supporting co-existence to a point where health services and education services are linked inextricably to a point of symbiotic existence. This approach acknowledges the contribution of education as a potential key driver of professional practice and health care improvements and emphasizes the need for continuing investment in education services.

Professional development

The current influence on effective management within the NHS has developed a culture of high expectations in relation to team and individual performance and has highlighted the need to review processes, structures, roles and responsibilities. The increasing demand on individuals to perform well within a climate of efficiency and effectiveness means that, for health professionals, there is a need to continually strive towards attaining and maintaining the highest performance standards. In essence the current approach to health care policy has raised the bar on both organizational and individual performance.

The DH has produced a plethora of literature relating to practice standards and continuing professional development (DH 2004a, 2005b, 2006a,b,c; Secretary of State for Health 2007) and professional regulation organizations have similarly demonstrated their commitment (HPC 2008a,c; NMC 2008b, 2006; GMC 2006). This signifies a collective approach to achieving and maintaining improved professional standards and developing an environment that is focused on teaching and learning.

The DH has set the scene and it is for individual NHS organizations and, in particular, NHS managers and educators to engage health care practitioners in professional development. Arguably, professional development is a process that benefits from a 'top down' approach in order to ensure quality processes and effective mentorship. Cathart *et al.* (2004) cite the longitudinal study on employee engagement conducted by the Gallop Organization. 'They discovered that talented employees need great managers' (Carthart *et al.* 2004, p. 396). Based on this finding, in order to encourage and support 'talent', it would be advisable to have sufficiently able managers in key roles. Although the relevance of the Harvard Business School (HBS) to the NHS might be questionable, it is notable that they take a similar view. The HBS discuss the concept of 'C performers', this term might imply average ability but interestingly is used by HBS to describe a manager of low ability. The HBS found that 'C performers':

'aren't good role models, coaches or mentors for others. Eighty percent of respondents in our survey said working for a low performer prevented them from learning, (and) kept them from making greater contributions to the organization' (HBS 2006, p. 114).

Interestingly, the HBS (2006) question the enormity of the level of impact on both employee talent pool and morale if such individuals each line manage or substantially influence ten people within an organization. Consideration of the potential scope of that influence within the NHS would suggest that under-performing managers should, as a minimum measure, be performance managed with the aim of improving outcomes for the individual, the staff they manage and ultimately for service users including patients. Within the perioperative environment, the term manager could be defined widely and applied equally to team leaders and clinical supervisors with the potential resultant effect magnified across the department.

Depending upon factors such as leadership style and level of experience, development of others in the form of delegation could prove problematic for some line managers as they may question the effectiveness of personally completing a task over the facilitation of others. They may potentially feel a loss of authority or feel de-skilled by delegation but, arguably, the responsibility of supporting others in new activities can in itself prove challenging and rewarding. Belbin (2004 p. 120) suggests, 'Some managers are as remarkable for what they refrain from doing as for what they do'. This approach would appear to define delegation as strategic and developmental rather than de-skilling or exploitative. Belbin (2004) advocates the benefit of identifying and delegating specific responsibilities that add value to team outcomes advocating;

'The skilled teamsman sets up others in appropriate team roles for which he prepares the ground by creating a void into which they can enter' (2004, p. 121).

This analogy offers a graphic depiction of the facilitation process. Within the perioperative setting, however, it may be interesting to indulge in semantics and exchange the word 'void' for platform or stage as the words theatres, stage and performance, when used in combination, conjure up a dramatic image of the facilitation process directing the spotlight on individual achievement. When delegating specific responsibilities to team members it is essential that the individual and other team members understand the purpose of that activity and its relevance to defined goals including organizational goals. In the current climate of 'choose and book'; a manager would be wise to define in what ways a delegated responsibility contributes to added value of patient services, acknowledging that 'Value is defined by the receivers . . . more than the givers' (Brockbank and Ulrich 2005, p. 11).

In consideration of the potential need to further develop individuals, NHS organizations need to ensure structure, consistency and equity in performance management systems and, when taking remedial action to manage performance, they should consider in what ways managerial or organizational actions or omissions may have impacted on performance outcomes. Roland *et al.* (2001) discuss a system for managing poor performing general practitioners (GPs). They describe a performance panel approach within which it is notable that decisions to instigate supportive improvement procedures are based on concerns raised rather than on routine performance monitoring. Arguably, the general practitioners, their associated teams and those individuals for whom the GPs represented a cause for concern, would have benefited from the pre-existence of a more structured, supportive and timely approach to performance development monitoring.

A report by the Chief Medical Officer 'Good doctors, safer patients' (DH 2006), the title of which succinctly identifies the first priority in performance development, was commissioned by the Secretary of State for Health following publication of the Shipman Inquiry; fifth report. In relation to public and professional attitudes the report acknowledged that:

'Both the public and doctors have firm views as to which aspects of practice can and should be assessed; these views are not very different' (DH 2006, p. xi)

In addition to clinical skills, issues of communication, involvement, dignity and respect were detailed as important to patients (DH 2006). The document offers 44 recommendations for achieving improvements, including developments in relation to the appraisal process.

The Government White Paper 'Trust, Assurance and Safety – The Regulation of Health Professionals in the 21st Century' (Secretary of State for Health 2007) addresses Regulation of the Health Professions in the wider context. The emphasis of this document similarly focuses on patient perceptions and aims to preserve trust, thus promoting effective relationships between patients and health professionals. The report offers proposals in relation to revalidation of registration and education and confirms support for the NHS appraisal process.

The NHS knowledge and skills framework and perioperative template system

Personal Development Reviews are central to staff development and therefore arguably central to organisational development in that they direct and record development activities and progress. The Introduction of Agenda for Change and with it the Knowledge and Skills Framework has established for the first time within the NHS a national performance review system that operates across the organization. The system 'provides a single, consistent, comprehensive and explicit framework on which to base review and development for all staff' (DH 2004c, p. 3). It aims to nurture a culture of performance development within the NHS and within that environment support individuals on a continuous basis to achieve the performance level required of their role. Its structures necessitate support and provision of opportunities for employees to assist their achievement including regular development review.

Knowledge and skills framework: *four things you need to know*

1. KSF scope and purpose

The DH (2004c) details application of the KSF system to be inclusive of a whole range of professional, technical, clerical and support service roles, and exclusive only of doctors, dentists and the most senior managers. The purpose is described to include the establishment of a uniform, structured approach to the development of individuals and teams, emphasizing support in terms of resources, and assistance for people to develop both within their current role and through a range of career pathways.

2. KSF dimensions

The KSF is described as comprising a range of dimensions or groups of objectives (DH 2004c). They include 'core dimensions', which are applicable to all roles for example the communication and health and safety dimensions and 'specific dimensions', which

are designed to support the individual requirements of some posts. Each dimension is available at four levels and all offer indicators which describe 'how knowledge and skills need to be applied at that level' (DH 2004c, p. 7). In addition, a range of examples of responsibilities or activities are offered through which the indicators can be met.

3. KSF outlines

The KSF (DH 2004c) enables the formation of outlines to support individual NHS roles. The outlines necessarily incorporate the six core dimensions that relate to key NHS objectives as reflected in the AfC National Agreement and a selection of specific or speciality dimensions that reflect the key responsibilities of a particular post. The appropriate level for the role is defined for each dimension, thus allowing organizations to demonstrate progression within career structures.

The inclusion of outline subsets accommodates preceptorship practitioners and newly promoted employees by defining a preliminary achievement level that reflects the 'basic knowledge and skills required from the outset in a post coupled with that needed after 12 months of development and support' (DH 2004c p. 26). In instances of promotion the dimension level required of the subset may be equal to that required of the immediately subordinate post, i.e. the level the individual was achieving before promotion.

A further advantage of the KSF is that it offers individuals the opportunity to develop above the level required for their current post.

'Career progression and development might take place by moving up levels in the same dimension or by adding on different dimensions as individuals move into new areas of work' (DH 2004c, p. 36).

For example, practitioners who are experienced in their roles and achieving all of their current role requirements as detailed in the KSF post outline may choose to discuss with their line manager opportunities to develop to a level above the requirements of their role in some key areas. This achievement would, of course, be evidenced and the benefit of this facility to individuals and organizations is that it assists both the reviewer and the reviewee to prepare towards promotional opportunities. Not all employees are interested, or continue to be interested, in career development. The DH (2004c) acknowledges this as an acceptable approach for some individuals,

'Provided that the individuals are able to apply their knowledge and skills to meet the demands of the post for which they are employed – which means they will be able to pass through the second gateway at the due time' (DH 2004c, p. 37).

Individuals preferring this option will, of course, continue to be subject to the AfC Personal Development Plan (PDP) process in order to assist development within their current role. The DH advises that, in these circumstances, the PDP is likely to 'focus on enabling the individual to maintain their current knowledge and skills and develop these to meet any changing requirements' (DH 2004c, p. 37).

4. The gateway phenomenon

The term 'gateway' is defined as 'an opening that can be closed by a gate' (*Oxford English Dictionary*, 2005, p. 375), which perhaps reflects why many practitioners approach the concept of AfC payband gateways with trepidation. Possibly, KSF discussions do not sufficiently emphasize that the gateway is expected to be open, particularly with sufficient preparation. Fortunately, a further definition is offered 'a means of entering somewhere or achieving something: the gateway to success' (*Oxford English Dictionary*, 2005, p. 375). This definition with its depiction of a gateway as a point on a journey and allusion to opportunities would seem more positive, progressive and pertinent to the AfC concept. A gate may, of course, be monitored by a gatekeeper and, in this instance, the role of gatekeeper falls to the PDP reviewer who holds responsibility to consider the gathered evidence and confirm whether the reviewee has right of passage in the form of a successfully achieved PDP. This in essence does no more than signify that the

individual is currently fulfilling the required elements of their role, at which point the gatekeeper will 'hold open the gate'.

The Agenda for Change paybands incorporate two gateways that act as pause points for confirmation of progress and link to pay progression. The 'Foundation Gateway' takes place no later than 12 months after an individual is appointed to a payband regardless of the pay point to which the individual is appointed. At the foundation gateway, an individual would be expected to meet the defined KSF outline subset levels as a minimum requirement. The DH (2004c) stipulates that

'At the second gateway the development review focuses on confirming that the individual is meeting the full demands of the post-as expressed in the NHS KSF post outline' (2004c, p. 24).

This statement does not, however, negate the fact that individuals should arguably be aiming to meet the full demands of the role before that time as consideration of the paybands would demonstrate that at the point of reaching the second gateway, individuals may have held a post for some 5–6 years.

The perioperative template discussion

In view of the vastness of the NHS and the incorporated roles, the KSF is defined by the DH (2004c, p. 5) as 'a broad generic framework . . . it does not describe the exact knowledge and skills that people need to develop'. The DH advises;

'The examples of application in the NHS KSF are designed as triggers to help this process but they are *not* the whole answer. The actual areas of application should be worked out for each post' (DH 2004c, p. 21).

In consideration of this inevitable limitation it may be valid to consider whether a co-existing framework with examples of perioperative knowledge and skills designed to link directly with the requirements of the dimension indicators could play a useful supporting role in assisting perioperative practitioners to measure and plan their learning and development. The following discussion summarized in Appendix I explores the potential benefits and constraints of such a system and offers a practical approach to how it might be implemented as demonstrated in Appendix II.

With the current focus on *personal* development plans, both reviewers and reviewees might initially recoil at the prospect of a KSF template system for perioperative roles, considering it a prescriptive approach to performance measurement objectives. The motivation to establish a perioperative template system (PTS) is, however, founded in economy, efficiency and standardization of processes. The PTS would aim to do no more than illustrate the dimension indicators in perioperative terms and assist the recording process.

It could be argued that the estimated time factors would be substantial should each organization and more likely each individual be required to interpret the KSF indicators in terms of specific roles. The proposed template approach would be linked inextricably to the existing KSF performance development system with the added advantage that it offers examples of activities and responsibilities that are specific to perioperative practice. The PTS would aim to operate in acceptance of the abundance of aspects that are key and common to the range of perioperative roles within NHS Trusts and to define those factors in terms of relevant examples of application. Most importantly, the PTS would offer a time-reduced and therefore cost-effective approach to interpreting the KSF within perioperative practice, thus affording individuals the maximum time to focus on the more personal task of directing their activities and contributing to team aims, thereby supporting their personal development. Contemplating the KSF Dimensions and their indicators, and interpreting them to enable identification and presentation of evidence towards a particular criterion, might be described as a skill in itself. In consideration of the diversity in the range and level of NHS roles, experience in this area could not be guaranteed. It is therefore questionable whether interpretation of the indicators in terms of an individual's role and responsibilities should be a prerequisite skill to a point where it is an essential, integral ingredient of all dimensions. It may, however, be equally questionable to deny employees the opportunity to exercise that skill albeit in a more limited and focused manner. Arguably experience in this area would be sufficiently explored in 'Core Dimension 2 Personal and People Development' (DH 2004c). This dimension supports responsibilities including defining learning objectives and measuring progress against criteria. For those with extended responsibilities in this area, 'Specific Dimension G1 Learning and Development' (DH 2004c) supports further development of these skills. Accepting this approach, the PTS would offer individuals sufficient scope to meet the indicators relating to their development and that of others.

There is limited information available at this stage on the implementation of the KSF, but a potential point of concern is equity in the level of evidence collected and presented to inform development review decisions. Arguably, in essence, evidence must be individual in order to be valid and traceable in order to facilitate monitoring processes. The DH (2004c p. 30) stipulates there must be a 'sufficiency of evidence' and that both the reviewer and the reviewee must;

'gather information on the individual's work against the NHS KSF outline for the post – this could be their own views of the individual's work, outputs from the individual's work (e.g. records, accounts) or be information from other people who have worked with the individual' (DH 2004c, p. 30).

In an attempt to support the KSF system and assist the development review process, the proposed PTS offers an optional system that would provide clear and specific perioperative examples of evidence that might be gathered and reviewed. The template would equally allow more experienced or innovative individuals amongst reviewers and reviewees to collect or request other forms of evidence that could be recorded within the PTS or the parallel system (Appendix III). In the first instance, however, examples of activities and evidence types in relation to perioperative roles would be available and afford both the reviewer and the reviewee more specific guidance and the confidence to commence the evidence gathering and recording process. Most essentially, the template would direct reviewers and reviewees alike to consider the wide range of potential activities in which perioperative practitioners might be involved.

It is intended that familiarity of both the reviewer and the reviewee with the PTS would optimize the time available for the development discussion and would facilitate consensual approval of directly observed or more common types of evidence and encourage detailed dialogue in exploration of more individual or complex evidence. Ultimately the discussion would specifically focus on personal evidence rather than on the general responsibilities of the role and would encourage involvement in activities designed to develop the individual to the upper limits of the role.

The system would aim to support the reviewer in their obligation to seek and ensure development opportunities for reviewees in that the appearance of a specific example of application might prove a helpful prompt for discussion. In this way the system would aim to minimize the instances where indicators may not be achieved due to lack of opportunity. It is intended that the PTS might also serve to assist both reviewers and reviewees to open up discussion to areas where an individual's performance may be below the expected level for the role. Supportive dialogue in relation to a predetermined example would afford both the reviewer and the reviewee confidence in the relevance and equity of the developmental discussion, in that the example would represent an accepted aspect of the role and one which the reviewee and other post holders could be expected to meet.

It is essential to note that reviewees would not be required to provide evidence of all the PTS examples listed at each review or even within a 12-month PDP cycle. The examples of application are intended to provide a selection of ways in which each indicator could be met. The specific examples for which evidence is to be gathered could be discussed and agreed between the reviewer and the reviewee within the initial PDP planning dialogue. The scope of the examples evidenced could, of course, be varied over the duration of the annual review or extended to PDPs in subsequent years. The ultimate decision as to what constitutes sufficient evidence to demonstrate meeting of the Outline Indicators would remain with the reviewer.

As a recommendation examples of application provided within the PTS would be subject to review as required in order to ensure that the types of evidence listed continue to reflect developments within perioperative practice and roles.

The process for recording evidence gathered and development review discussions and outcomes would remain flexible within the boundaries of Trust or regional documentation. The PTS would, however, aim to support the process by providing a record of the evidence presented and considered at the development review. The PTS would not, in itself, hold the gathered evidence, but could assist audit processes by recording traceable evidence on which development decisions had been based.

Conclusion

There is currently a determined 'Agenda for Change' in the NHS, a fundamental review of what, when, where and how services are delivered. The DH aims to reform health service delivery (DH 2001) (DH 2005a) (DH 2005c) and the influence and intervention of education would appear to be essential to the implementation of the modernization agenda. In order to achieve the required improvements, DH and professional policy (DH 2006b; GMC 2006; HPC 2008a,c; NMC 2008b) have focused on professional development and effective mentorship as an essential resource and mechanism in achieving quality improvements and arguably the development review system is central to this process. The DH (2004c) acknowledges that essential service improvements, patient safety and public confidence will be best achieved and supported by investment in a continually developing workforce. To this purpose, the DH has implemented a review of professional regulation processes (Secretary of State for Health 2007), emphasizing the responsibilities of regulatory bodies to provide for, and monitor, educational needs of registrants and the responsibility of individuals to provide evidence of fitness to practise to support professional revalidation.

The DH has invested for the first time in a uniform staff development structure within the NHS that is organization wide with the flexibility to support the development of individuals in specific roles. For the multitude of employees it provides for, the KSF represents a generic structure for support and performance measurement and a framework for the development of individuals both within their roles and within new career pathways. The structure simultaneously assists registered practitioners towards their responsibility to demonstrate competent practice and continuing professional development as required by professional regulation organizations.

The proposed Perioperative Template System (Appendix II, III) would aim to assist that requirement, making the KSF indicators more accessible to perioperative employees by interpreting them in perioperative terms.

The PTS would aim to facilitate this without inhibiting the initiative and innovation of individuals in interpreting the KSF indicators and gathering evidence to demonstrate personal development.

The KSF (DH 2004c) incorporates structures and processes to assist the transition of health care employees towards, and through, the AfC payband gateways as a natural consequence of supportive and directed development. A possible measurement of its success would therefore be the optimum development of individuals at the earliest point post-foundation gateway.

The development of the KSF national structure has created a firm foundation towards standardization of the development review system, but arguably a framework with the scope of the KSF is open to both local and individual interpretation and there is a potential for standards to vary. The success of the KSF is therefore dependent upon the commitment of NHS managers to ensure the system is implemented in a manner that is supportive, equitable and robust. Arguably, systems audit as an intrinsic and essential factor is necessary to assure quality of processes.

Accepting this, it is expected that the introduction of the KSF across the NHS will facilitate demonstrable improvements to the opportunities available and development experienced by NHS employees which is likely to enable the provision of value-added services, with the ultimate test of quality being measured in terms of increased patient safety, improved patient experience and positive public perceptions of health care.

Appendix I Frequently asked questions

Question 1 Is the perioperative template system intended to replace the NHS KSF?

Answer No, the PTS is not intended to replace the NHS KSF, it closely adheres to the KSF core and specific dimension indicators and interprets these in terms of perioperative roles, offering relevant examples of how they may be achieved.

Question 2 The PTS appears to be quite prescriptive. Does it allow for *personal* development and individual interpretation of the evidence to be collected?

Answer Yes, the PTS offers a semi-standardized approach by identifying a range of perioperative examples of application. Equally it allows for additional personalized evidence to be provided in support of the indicators and 'free text' in the parallel system.

Question 3 Does the PTS allow for individuals to set individual objectives for the reviewee?

Answer Yes, the PTS provides scope for reviewers to define individual objectives for reviewees and allows reviewees the opportunity to demonstrate their skill in objective setting within 'Core Dimension 2: Personal and People Development'.

Question 4 Will the standardized format inhibit the free flow of discussion during the review and prevent the reviewer from making their own decisions?

Answer No, the semi-standardized format and recording system encourages some standardization in the evidence collected and measured and therefore allows more time for discussion of more individual objectives and evidence within the PDP meeting.

Question 5 How would the PTS help a reviewer to review the development of an individual who was perceived to be under-performing?

Answer The PTS is likely to direct the discussion towards the specific areas of practice that are the causes of concern. Predetermined examples would assist in advising and reassuring the reviewee that the objectives are expected of all individuals within the role.

Question 6 Is a system that incorporates tick boxes more open to misuse as reviewers who are not committed to the process could approve all evidence listed by the reviewee without full consideration?

Answer If individuals are not committed to the development review process, any system would be open to misuse including the NHS KSF. The PTS tick boxes offers assistance in getting started and the parallel system provides a recording system for more experienced individuals. In order to ensure quality processes it is recommended that the process be audited, and the level of documentation is designed to assist audit processes.

Appendix II Illustrative Example of the Perioperative Template System

Core Dimension 3 Health Safety and Security Level 2

KSF indicators	Examples of application: Indicators may be achieved by involvement in the following types of activities	Annual development Review Number/Date		
		1	2	3
		10.4.08	11.9.08	15.1.09

(a)	Manages risks in patient transfer. . . .
(b)	Utilizes waterlow score. . . . . .
(c)	Has attended mandatory training sessions
Undertakes work activities consistent with: – legislation, policies and procedures – the assessment and management of risk	Has attended essential training Has completed all relevant perioperative medical device competency forms Conducts safety checks and prepares equipment for operative procedures Effectively completes patient perioperative checks Demonstrates an understanding of Health & Safety Legislation and Trust and Perioperative Care policies and procedures and guidelines for practice Including Demonstrates safe practice in relation to Trust and perioperative policies, procedures and guidelines for practice. Protects others from immediate risks in the perioperative environment Reports any noted risks to the appropriate person Understands the risk assessment process Adheres to documented risk assessments Suggests an area of practice that would benefit from audit Contributes to audit of safe practice Conducts audit of safe practice Completes electronic Trust untoward incident or near miss form Record of learning from Health & Safety Seminar Record of learning from shadowing Risk Lead Written assignment/article on Health and Safety Practice **Reviewee examples include:** Reflection on untoward incident Evidence from HPC Portfolio
(d)	Cares for patients in emergency situations for example. . . .
(e)	Aware of process for reporting. . . .
(f)	Advises new members of staff on importance of. . . . .
(a) (b) (c) (d) (e) (f)	Evidence gathered and reviewed to support the above: Mandatory Training Record

Appendix II (*cont.*)

Core Dimension 3 Health Safety and Security Level 2

KSF indicators	Examples of application: Indicators may be achieved by involvement in the following types of activities	Annual development Review Number/Date		
		1	2	3
		10.4.08	11.9.08	15.1.09
	Review of Speciality Equipment Competency Folder Copies of Attendance & Learning Records from Audit Day Training Sessions Reviewer's observations of reviewee's performance in patient care activities Infection control audit form completed by reviewee Recently completed untoward incident form Reflection of Untoward Incident completed by reviewee Record of learning from Tissue Viability module Record of learning from Infection Control study day			

Appendix III Illustrative Example of the Perioperative Template System

Core Dimension 2 Personal and People Development Level 4

KSF indicators	Evidence of achievement: The following examples represent traceable activities the reviewee has been involved in. Evidence of these examples can be provided on request	Annual development Review Number/Date		
		1	2	3
		10.4.08	11.9.08	15.1.09
(a) evaluates the currency and sufficiency of own knowledge and pratice against the KSF outline for the post and identifies own development needs and interests	This document and accompanying completed PDP form. Determines above in relation to organisational and departmental objectives and current role requirements as discussed with reviewer/line manager.	✓ ✓	✓ ✓	✓ ✓
(b) develops and agrees own personal development plan with feedback from others	Contributes to PDP discussion with reviewer/line manager Suggests areas for own development e.g. C&G 9295 Certificate in Adult Learning support, Mentorship in Practice. Defines how above learning will support role and enhance achievements (Learning objectives available).	✓ ✓ ✓	✓	✓ ✓
(c)	Utilized information from C&G 9295......			✓
(d)	Discusses records of reflective practice with......	✓		
(e)	Devises Development Programmes to support...	✓		
(f) actively promotes the workplace as a learning environment encouraging everyone to learn from each other and from external good practice	Provision of monthly Audit Day Perioperative Development Programme. Ensures opportunities for staff members to share information and update knowledge on health & safety policies and practices, medical device training and other development issues for example mentorship updates, NVQ (perioperative care) workshops	✓	✓	✓
	(Copy Programmes, attendance and evaluation forms available). Ensure adequate number of trained mentors in perioperative areas (Training records available)	✓		
	Ensures allocation of mentors for pre and post-registration students. Implemented weekly mentor allocation record (records available)	✓	✓	
	Provision and monitoring of learning resources e.g. library books reference documents	✓		
	Provision of protected learning time and 'student status' for individuals on development programmes.	✓		
(g)	Procured Perioperative Moving and Handling DVDs	✓		
(h)	Ensures inclusive opportunities to develop for example...	✓		

REFERENCES

Belbin, R. M. (2004). *Management Teams*, 2nd edn Elsevier, pp. 120, 121.

Brockbank, W. & Ulrich, D. (2005). *The HR Value Proposition*, Harvard Business School Press, p. 11.

Cathart, D., Jeska, S., Karnas, J., Miller, S., Pechacek, J. & Rheault, L. (2004). Span of Control Matters. *Journal of Nursing Administration*, **34** (9), 395–9.

Department of Health (2001). *Building a safer NHS for patients: Implementing an organization with a memory* April, p. 6.

Department of Health (2004a). *Modernizing Medical Careers* April, p. 1.

Department of Health (2004b). *Choose & Book Patient's Choice of Hospital and Booked Appointment* August, pp. 3–4, 7, 9, 11–12.

Department of Health (2004c). *The NHS Knowledge and Skills Framework (NHS KSF) and the Development Review Process* October, pp. 3, 5–7, 11, 21, 23–4, 26, 30, 36–7, 57–61, 178–82.

Department of Health (2005a). *Creating a Patient-led* NHS Delivering the NHS Improvement Plan DH London, March, pp. 3–10.

Department of Health (2005b). *Anaesthesia Practitioner Curriculum Framework* London, June, pp. 2, 4.

Department of Health (2005c). *A Short Guide to NHS Foundation Trusts* November, p. 1.

Department of Health (2006a). *The Curriculum Framework for the Surgical Care Practitioner* London, March.

Department of Health (2006b). *Good Doctors, Safer Patients* July, pp. vi, vii, xi, 194.

Department of Health (2006c). *Modernizing Nursing Careers* September, p. 3.

Department of Health (2009). *Valuing People Now: A Three-Year Strategy for People with Learning Disabilities* London, January, pp. 24, 26–7, 30.

Ellis, H. (2009). Marie Curie: discoverer of radium. *Journal of Perioperative Practice*, **19** (1), p. 36.

General Medical Council (2006). *Good Medical Practice Regulating doctors ensuring good medical practice* London, p. 14.

Harvard Business Essentials (2006). *Performance Management*, Harvard Business School Press, p. 114.

Health Professions Council (2008a) *Your Guide to Our Standards for Continuing Professional Development*, April, pp. 1–3.

Health Professions Council (2008b). *Standards of conduct, performance and ethics* July, pp. 1, 5, 11, 12, 15.

Health Professions Council (2008c). *Standards of Proficiency, Operating Department Practitioners* October, pp. 6, 8, 9, 10.

Nightingale F (2006). *Notes on Nursing.* Tempus Publishing, pp. 52–4, 54, 99, 137, 154, 156.

Nursing & Midwifery Council (2006). *Standards to support learning and assessment in practice* August, pp. 7, 8, 10, 11, 14, 20–3.

Nursing & Midwifery Council (2008a). *The Code: Standards of Conduct, Performance and Ethics for Nurses and Midwives* London, May, pp. 1–2.

Nursing & Midwifery Council (2008b). *Standards to Support Learning and Assessment in Practice: NMC Standards for Mentors, Practice Teachers and Teachers.* London, July, pp. 1, 6–8, 11, 13, 16.

Oxford English Dictionary (2005). 10th edn Oxford University Press, p. 375.

Pell, J. P. & Smith, G. C. S., (2003). Parachute use to prevent death and major trauma related to gravitational challenge: systematic review of randomised controlled trials. *British Medical Journal*, **327**, 1459–60.

Perioperative Care Collaborative (2007). *Position Statement: The Role and Responsibilities of the Advanced Scrub Practitioner* Association of Perioperative Practitioners Harrogate, pp. 2–4.

Roland, M., Copek, M., Freedman, R., Wearne, M. (2001). Catch a falling star. *Health Service Journal*, **111** (5745), 30–1.

Secretary of State for Health, (2007). *Trust, Assurance and Safety: The Regulation of Health Professionals in the 21st Century* London, The Stationery Office, pp. 6, 39, 69.

World Alliance for Patient Safety (2008). *Implementation Manual Surgical Safety Checklist, Safe Surgery Saves Lives* Switzerland, World Health Organization. 1st edn May, p. 2.

14

Equipment procurement: a purchaser's guide for theatre managers

Peter Norman

Key Learning Points

- Understand the models used when considering purchases
- Appreciate the value of differing actors in the purchasing process
- Enhance effectiveness in purchasing for theatres by engaging more effectively with the purchasing team

Introduction

There are many sayings to do with looking after finances. Two are are 'Look after the pennies and the pounds will look after themselves' and 'Penny wise pound foolish'. While the first saying has truth, it can often distract you from the second.

This chapter is intended to provide some advice and guidance on how to look after an operating theatre budget and get the most for each pound. It is often a lot easier to save money from current spending than it is to get new funding for improved patient care, and it can also be more rewarding.

Purchasing has grown in recent years from a clerical function to a strategic function (Ellram & Carr 1994), becoming a leading profession in business. The big supermarkets, car manufacturers and service providers – transport, leisure and banking – all rely heavily on their ability to specify, buy and manage their goods and services to give them a competitive and leading edge in the market. Similar to accountants and surveyors, purchasing professionals build on their academic qualifications and further develop their specialist knowledge, experience, tools and techniques in purchasing and supply. The profession is represented by its own institute, the Chartered Institute of Purchasing and Supply (2008).

Purchasing is not just about buying at the lowest cost or 'face' price, it is about whole life costing – which means the total cost of products or services across their lifetime (Whole Life Costing Forum 2008).

That total cost includes the cost of purchase plus the time taken to draw up the business case or justifying the need:

- writing the specification: often including input from a team of appropriate specialists
- obtaining quotations: which can take up to four months and cost up to £20 000
- putting the purchase in place: which can include specialist fitting or training
- consumable costs: which often are more over time than the initial purchase
- running costs: for running and maintain equipment
- disposal costs: which, because of new regulations, are often built into the purchase price, and the cost to the environment such as air miles, deforestation, ethical considerations (e.g. slave and child labour).

Core Topics in Operating Department Practice: Leadership and Management, ed. Brian Smith, Paul Rawling, Paul Wicker and Chris Jones. Published by Cambridge University Press. © Cambridge University Press 2010.

These are just some of the issues to be considered when making a purchase decision. Purchasing can be used to have broader societal or environmental benefits and impacts (Walker *et al.* 2008).

Sales and marketing

To understand how to buy well it is important to understand how you are 'sold' to by suppliers (Ford 2002). Suppliers to the healthcare market are no different to suppliers in other markets as they are there to sell you their products. They take into consideration a number of issues. What is a profitable area to be in? How difficult is it to enter the market? Do we have the product or service to compete? Can we break in, stay in and make a sustainable profit? If a positive answer can be given to these questions, they now have to decide the best route to market.

In many cases the supplier will have to develop a product (e.g. a piece of equipment) that they believe is better than their competition. This is often done by developing new or additional 'features and benefits' that are said to be better than the alternatives available. This gives them advantage over their competitors (Porter 1998).

Features and benefits are a standard part of any sales representative's presentation. If you buy a DVD player from the High Street, the sales person will point out all the additional features that will help you record easily or fast forward to a specific place or remember where you last stopped watching – all additional features and all to 'benefit' you. Often these additional features do not necessarily bring any actual benefit to the customer (ask yourself how often you use the additional 'gadgets' you have been sold), but the purpose is to set the product apart from alternatives or to justify an additional or premium price.

Once suppliers have their product, they then 'segment' their customer base (Cooil *et al.* 2007) and identify the people who can make or influence the purchase decision in some way. In carrying out this segmentation, they can identify certain key audiences and craft their sales presentation accordingly.

In most cases, there is a decision-making unit (Robinson *et al.* 1967), which could consist of the team of specialists mentioned above, and the supplier's sales team will target this team and each member specifically with the messages, the features and benefits that they want to hear. This will be delivered over a range of media, for example through meetings, presentations, conferences, sponsorship, training events, bursaries and so on. A visit to the conference of the National Association of Theatre Nurses will give you some idea of the money that is spent in targeting messages in addition to the company representatives who visit the workplace bringing their latest product news.

Suppliers will concentrate their efforts on making the potential customer want their product. Once they have done that, they will talk price and help the customer find ways to afford and justify the purchase. The pricing of products is a complex area and, as discussed above, it is not just the initial purchase price but the whole life cost. All these costs need to be identified and evaluated.

Remember, a supplier will want to influence the theatre manager and the clinicians to have a preference for their products over others. This is understandable for the supplier, as it is for clinical staff. Most people have different tastes and preferences in their home life but in theatres a more pragmatic approach must be taken to ensure that products are truly evaluated on the basis of quality, efficacy (Does it do what it is supposed to do? Is it effective?), availability, cost and so on. It is important that clinical preference (Cox *et al.* 2005, Zheng *et al.* 2006) is not the only parameter for selecting the best product or piece of equipment and that an open and robust sourcing exercise takes place and the alternatives are assessed and evaluated properly.

Know the theatre's spend

Key to getting the best out of a budget is knowing the spend. This can be found by meeting with the assigned accountant and reviewing the budget and spend detail. Ask for spend information for the past 12 months and sort it by spend type (equipment purchase, consumables, services, maintenance), by supplier and, if possible, by product – this is known as a 'spend cube'. Once this has been done, it is possible to analyse and categorize the spend in many useful and informative ways.

It may be that the information is hard to sort and review. This may be because of poor coding. Your organization's finance and supply functions will have a coding system to identify and charge products and services. This will include a budget code, an item code and a supplier code, and it is by these codes that the spend information can be sorted. It is important, therefore, to follow the coding structure and avoid using 'bucket' or 'dump' codes. The information obtained from the accountant often reflects the information provided through the coding of orders. Raise this issue with the accountant and familiarize yourself with and follow the correct coding practice.

Pareto analysis (the 80/20 rule)

A good way to begin to understand a unit's spend is to carry out at Pareto analysis. The Italian Vilfredo Pareto observed that, regardless of the country studied, a small portion of the population controlled most of the wealth, and this concept was adopted by business writer Joseph Juran (1964). This observation led to the Pareto rule (or curve), the general principles of which hold in a wide range of situations. In purchasing and supply, the Pareto rule usually holds for items purchased, number of suppliers, items held in inventory and many other aspects. The Pareto curve is often called the 80/20 rule or ABC analysis.

This can be illustrated with a home budget that lists expenditure and the number of 'suppliers' (Table 14.1). The actual amounts filled in column 3 would probably demonstrate that about 70% to 80% of spend (mortgage and utilities) goes with possibly two or three suppliers whereas 20%–30% (the rest)

Table 14.1 A home budget

Expenditure	Suppliers	Value
Mortgage	1	
Utility bills	1 or 2	
House 'equipment'	3	
Rates	1	
Food	8	

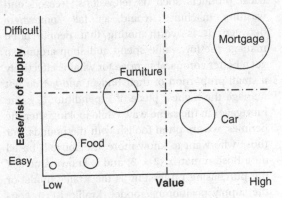

Figure 14.1 Mapping supply against value for a home budget. The size of each circle represents amount of spend.

goes with 10 or 12. Hence, 80% of the household spend is with 20% of its suppliers.

Spend profile

Once spend is sorted into categories, it is possible to begin to consider how important each category is and/or how easily available it is. More often than not, simple economics dictates that a product or service that has high demand but few to supply has a higher market price, whereas a product or service that has a low demand with high supply has a lower price. A new medical technology (equipment or drug) owned by one supplier and that is high in demand will be expensive. Polythene bin liners, mass produced, will be relatively cheap.

Consider the home budget and map out the categories of spend on the two axes (Fig. 14.1). Certain things will be regular items of expenditure, such as food and drink, newspapers or petrol, and these will be bought from the local shop/supermarket or be delivered. These items would be in the bottom left corner of the matrix as they are low in value and there is an abundance of supply. The largest proportion of expenditure is usually the house (mortgage), the car and all insurance payments. All of these are likely to fall towards the top right. Electrical products such as televisions, freezers and washing machines would all fall somewhere between. It is worth noting that people often manage the low value spend and shop around to get a better comparable price for what is effectively a small proportion of their budget and yet do not manage the highest piece of expenditure (e.g. the mortgage) in the same way. While looking after the pennies, we are often foolish with the pounds. For those who want to know more, the above is based on a Boston matrix (2 × 2) and is known amongst the purchasing profession as the Kraljic model or the supply positioning model (Kraljic 1983), contrasting the supply risk and profit impact of products/services.

Once an analysis of this type has been carried out, it is possible to start considering how to deal with suppliers in each category. For those where there is an abundance of supply, it is advisable to look to an integrated delivery service with a low 'acquisition' cost (the list price plus normal incidental costs to acquire the item including preparation, transportation and installation). The days of travelling from shop to shop in search of the lowest priced loaf or bag of sugar are past and now one-stop shopping is the norm and this may even be done online and delivered. This is often the choice because time lost is more 'costly' than the money saved. This 'time' would be better used in considering what the best mortgage is. All of this is true in theatres.

As well as the above, it is important to consider how costs may be reduced through reduced use. The obvious ones for a theatre are reducing the use of electricity, hitting two targets: spend reduction and environmental impact.

Working with the supply manager

The discussion above gives a flavour of what should be considered when managing a theatre budget but there is more to it than that.

All big hospitals have a supply or procurement manager and the theatre manager should get to know him or her. The role of the supply manager is to carry out the analysis above across all the expenditure of the organization. If this has been done properly, it is highly likely that theatre manager and supply manager will already have contacts as the latter will want to know all about the theatres as they have a high level of spend: the Pareto analysis again.

A good supply manager will:

- understand the organizations spend profile and will have strategies to get best value for that spend: this will be done by working with key decision makers and groups
- have good systems and procedures in place to manage the low-level expenditure items effectively: this is often done through the introduction of ward materials' management or top up with a focus on getting the lowest acquisition cost (cost of ordering the product, receiving it and getting it on the shelf for use)
- understand the high areas of expenditure and working with clinical colleagues and accountants to specify and agree the right products and evaluating their efficacy in use
- understand and take into account the organization's governance requirements (standing orders and financial instructions), procurement legislation (European Union regulations and UK law; Business in Partnership 2008) and health and safety requirements
- ensure that relevant health and safety issues are taken into account during purchase and installation (e.g. electrical checking, fire retardant properties).

This is a small sample of what procurement does. Procurement is a rapidly growing profession, both in its importance and in its influence in organizations. That said, one of the basic and most important roles of the supply manager will be to help the theatre manager to draw up and communicate his or her requirements, most often done through a detailed specification (Ramsay 1991). As well as improving the buying price, it is possible to negotiate additional services such as training, free product or improved warranty terms.

Some leading NHS Trusts have full-time clinical staff working closely with procurement staff. These people are known nationally as clinical procurement specialists (CPSs) and their job is to work effectively between clinical and procurement staff. They ensure that clinical requirements for products and services are properly specified and evaluated to ensure the most cost-effective products are identified and supplied. The CPSs often work with their clinical colleagues and establish standard products to be used across all wards and departments. They do an excellent job.

The specification: lead do not be led

This chapter began with how products and services are developed and promoted: new, improved products, with additional features and benefits, sold at a premium price. It is important, therefore, to identify specific needs and develop a personal specification to meet those needs and not to work in isolation. Consultation with other theatres (and other organizations) will identify what they use; the supply manager can help in doing this. The more a theatre's specification is developed in line with one particular supplier's product the more the theatre will be tied into that product and the higher the overall cost that is likely to be incurred. The more general the specification, the more competition there will be and the more likely it is that a lower price will be achieved. A specification should contain the features that are needed not the 'nice to haves'. Not only is it bad procurement to write a specification that may unnecessarily preclude suppliers it may be illegal under English law.

The price paid

Everyone is a buyer. Most are good buyers. So when it has been decided what is needed and the specification has been developed and sent out to market, it is then the time to consider the price that should be paid. This is done by considering other products and comparing their quality and relative price, the size of 'our' business (we might be buying a lot) and many factors.

For light relief, a price list is given for a product with variations in price with quantity purchased:

1–10: 100p
10–20: 80p
21–30: 60p
31–40: 40p
41+: 20p.

What should be paid for 20? The price list dictates, or suggests, that the price is 80p and that is what most will pay. Some people would look to pay 60p, maybe through some 'hard nose' negotiations with the salesperson. But consider this: the first batch of product (1–10) is 100p each: so that is equivalent to 10 at £1, or £10. The second batch is £8. Take the cost of the first batch of 10 from the second batch of ten and there is a difference of £2. Divide that £2 by the second batch of ten and you have a price of 20p each. The trick is to try and buy the second batch of ten at the 'marginal' price. It takes a while to understand this at face value but it becomes clear when you understand how suppliers price and sell their goods based on fixed and marginal costs.

Another 'tool' in the procurement kit is to consider the cost of making the product. This is called product price analysis (Lysons & Gillingham 2003). It can be done formally by requesting a full breakdown of costs for manufacturing a product and its cost to supply and maintain. This understanding is very useful when contesting price increases resulting from, say, a rise in oil and, therefore, plastics prices. It also helps in understanding the true cost as opposed to the market or brand value. Just recently, there was a television advert for a large supermarket advertising one of the 'top two' cola drinks at £1.50 (half price) for two litres. However, if this item is product re-engineered and the branding element discounted, its constituent costs are primarily water plus sugar syrup in a plastic bottle. Consumers may wish to pay for other factors such as brand or nice aesthetics or design in their home life but when spending public money managers need to take a more pragmatic and sensible approach. Further explanation of price tools will not be given here, but the above should demonstrate that there is a lot more to understanding 'price'.

The cost of acquisition

As well as the costs identified and outlined above, there is also the cost of acquisition. These are the costs incurred to identify, specify, source, contract, purchase, deliver and pay.

The cost for the process of placing, receiving and paying for one order alone by a large organization is estimated to be in the region of £40–70. Consider, therefore, placing an order for a piece of stationery for £10. The total costs will be more in the region of £50.

As highlighted above, a good supply manager will understand the spend profile of a department and will identify the freely available low-cost products and will put arrangements in place to ensure an integrated and dependable supply system that has the lowest acquisition cost. The car manufacturing industry, for example, uses 'just in time' methodology (Karlsson & Norr 1994) to keep the cost to the absolute minimum. This method ensures that supplies are not ordered (and paid for) until they are needed – just in time.

The main method used in the NHS to minimize these costs is materials management (Caridi & Cigolini 2002) or 'top up'. This is a system similar to that used in supermarkets to replenish stock and is used in most wards and departments now. Stock levels are pre-agreed by departmental managers and are maintained by stores, theatre or housekeeping staff. The process is set to help to maintain the most optimum stock levels and, more importantly, the most cost-effective supply route. In the main, products supplied via this route will be from a major one-stop distributor such as NHS Supply Chain (nww.nhssupplychain.nhs.uk).

As well as reduced acquisition costs, using a supply system such as materials management or equipment library (Audit Commission 1996) will ensure continuity of supply and that products and equipment are available and ready for use when they are needed. Again, the supply manager can help and advise on what is best for a particular department.

Collaboration

The NHS has seen many changes since the mid 1990s and many of these changes have been to do with competition and collaboration. These changes affect procurement as there have also been many changes to the NHS 'supply' infrastructure – primarily around centralizing and decentralizing the service. While this may continue to change, it is still true that there are real benefits to be had through collaboration. The more colleagues with a similar spend profile can join together and agree standard specifications and supply routes, the stronger they will become as a buyer or buying group.

There are many levels where collaboration can happen (Bakker *et al.* 2008) but the main place to start is at home within the hospital or Trust. Compare going out to market for several types of infusion pump from several suppliers, with several lots of consumables and several lots of training, storage, cleaning and maintenance, with going out once for one standard pump with standard consumables. Then imagine that equipment being bought and held in one place, cleaned and maintained and delivered only when needed. One standard pump would mean better training and understanding and reduced clinical risk, as accidents often happen through people being unfamiliar with equipment. This seems common sense, but a look around a hospital will show how much the equipment differs from ward to ward or department. Often equipment has a range of additional features and benefits, but are these extras necessary?

As well as local collaboration, there are wider NHS collaborative groups or purchasing arrangements that can be used, such as NHS Supply Chain, and also National Framework Agreements put in place by the NHS Purchasing and Supply Agency (www.pasa.nhs.uk). Both are part of the NHS and access to their agreements is free.

There are also collaborative arrangements put in place at a local level within health authority boundaries (collaborative procurement organizations: confederations and hubs) or across specialties such as cardiac and paediatric care. There are also collaborations across public sector organizations for buying common items such as recycled paper, energy or travel. The supply manager will know more.

Supplier representatives

This chapter has been quite adversarial in setting apart the buyer from the seller in this competition or power struggle (Cox 1999) to maintain margin or improve or reduce the purchase price. This should not be the way we do business. It is the suppliers who work to understand patient and clinician needs and make products and services to meet them. It is suppliers who are innovative and who develop and create better solutions to problems – the healthcare sector needs them and they are very important to hospitals and patients. Collaborating and communicating with suppliers has been shown to be beneficial for innovation and for bringing environmental benefits into the supply chain (Phillips *et al.* 2007, Vachon & Klassen 2008).

This leads to the suggestion that Trust purchasers should work with suppliers but on their own terms. Clinical procurement specialists are one way to improve the way Trusts source and evaluate products (ensuring efficacy in use – does it do what it says it does?) and another way is through product-evaluation teams. These teams work across wards and departments, together with procurement and finance colleagues, in identifying common equipment and products and ensuring the best-value products are selected and supplied. Remember there are real benefits in standardizing when negotiating with suppliers and there is real power when a Trust has the ability to change or switch product en masse.

By having such a group of specialists, the purchaser is able to target areas of spend and invite suppliers to come in and present to the group on what its members are looking for and not on what the suppliers are looking to sell. It also helps the sales people to concentrate on putting their efforts into where they are more likely to sell on a more sustainable footing and helps to bring in new innovations. Many Trusts now have a 'reps' policy which dictates that supplier representatives will not be allowed to visit wards or be seen by clinical staff unless they have visited the supplies department first to outline the purpose of their visit. By doing this, it may be decided that it is more appropriate for the supplier representative to present to the evaluation team, where a proper evaluation will be carried out (including current and future supply issues), rather than visiting each theatre or ward. These teams can also look at the life costing of equipment and consumables as there are cases of equipment being sold to one department at a knock-down price only for another department to pay excessive running or consumable costs.

This chapter is intended to give insight into some of the complexities of procurement. The main advice is to understand the spend. A manager should work with colleagues in supplies and finance to understand and get the best out of his or her budget and should collaborate to obtain a wider understanding, remembering that there is strength in numbers. Suppliers are not the enemy but they are there to do a job: selling their products or services. So, a manager needs to understand what is needed, to articulate that need through a good specification and to work with suppliers to get the best, most cost-effective solution in an organized way on the manager's terms.

REFERENCES

Audit Commission (1996). *Goods for Your Health*. London: Audit Commission.

Bakker, E., Walker, H., Schotanus, F. & Harland, C. (2008). Choosing an organizational form: the case of collaborative procurement initiatives. *International Journal of Procurement Management*, **1**, 297–317.

Business in Partnership (2008). http://www.bipsolutions.com/ (accessed 28 July 2008).

Caridi, M. & Cigolini, R. (2002). Improving materials management effectiveness: a step towards agile enterprise. *International Journal of Physical Distribution and Logistics Management*, **32**, 556–576.

Chartered Institute of Purchasing and Supply (2008). http://www.cips.org/ (accessed 28 July 2008).

Cooil, B., Aksoy, L. & Keiningham, T. (2007). Approaches to customer segmentation. *Journal of Relationship Marketing*, **6**, 9–39.

Cox, A. (1999). Power, value and supply chain management. *Supply Chain Management: An International Journal*, **4**, 167–175.

Cox, A., Chicksand, D. & Ireland, P. (2005). Sub-optimality in NHS sourcing in the UK: demand-side constraints on supply-side improvement. *Public Administration*, **83**, 367–392.

Ellram, L.M. & Carr, A. (1994). Strategic purchasing: a history and review of the literature. *International Journal of Purchasing and Materials Management*, Spring, 130–138.

Ford, D. (2002). *Understanding Business Marketing and Purchasing*. London: International Thomson.

Juran, J.M. (1964). *Managerial Breakthrough*. New York: McGraw-Hill.

Karlsson, C. & Norr, N. (1994). Total effectiveness in a just-in-time system. *International Journal of Operations and Production Management*, **14**, 46–65.

Kraljic, P. (1983). Purchasing must become supply management. *Harvard Business Review*, Sept–Oct, 109–117.

Lysons, K. & Gillingham, M. (2003). *Purchasing and Supply Chain Management*. London: Financial Times Management.

Phillips, W., Knight, L., Caldwell, N. & Warrington, J. (2007). Policy through procurement: the introduction of digital signal process (DSP) hearing aids into the English NHS. *Health Policy*, **80**, 77–85.

Porter, M.E. (1998). *Competitive Advantage: Creating and Sustaining Superior Performance*. New York: The Free Press.

Ramsay, J. (1991). Purchase specifications and profit performance. *International Journal of Physical Distribution and Logistics Management*, **21**, 34–41.

Robinson, P.J., Farris, C.W. & Wind, Y. (1967). *Industrial Buying and Creative Marketing*. Boston, MA: Allyn and Bacon.

Vachon, S. & Klassen, R.D. (2008). Environmental management and manufacturing performance: the role of collaboration in the supply chain. *International Journal of Production Economics*, **111**, 299–315.

Walker, H., diSisto, L. & McBain, D. (2008). Drivers of environmental supply chain practices: lessons from the public and private sectors. *Journal of Purchasing and Supply Management*, **14**, 69–85.

Whole Life Costing Forum (2008). *Whole Life Costing*; http://www.wlcf.co.uk/ (accessed 28 July 2008).

Zheng, J.R., Bakker, E., Knight, L. *et al.* (2006). A strategic case for e-adoption in healthcare supply chains. *International Journal of Information Management*, **26**, 290–301.

15

The reflective practitioner in perioperative settings

Anne Jones

Key Learning Points
- Understand the concept of reflective practice
- Explore the role of reflection in practice
- Use critical incident analysis as a basis for reflection

Introduction

In recent years, healthcare provision has changed significantly. It is with a degree of certainty that we can assume change will continue, as society undergoes progress and transformation. The rapid transformation has, and will continue to have, a direct impact on the role and function of all healthcare practitioners. Evolutionary history teaches that all organisms must adapt with their environment or die, and that organisms developing a feature that helps them to succeed in their environment prosper at the expense of those who do not (Handy 1989).

The changing environment in healthcare follows national direction as set out in the current government's policies. These were first outlined in the White Paper *The New NHS: Modern, Dependable* (Department of Health 1997), followed by the strategic framework presented in *The NHS Plan* (Department of Health 2000). These policies presented the vision for the NHS in the twenty-first century. More recently, further challenges in the reform journey within the NHS are presented in *High Quality Care for All: NHS Next Stage Review Final Report* (Department of Health 2008). This document recognizes that to enable the reforms articulated within it to be implemented there needs to be corresponding changes to the planning, education and training of the healthcare workforce. There is emphasis on the importance of team-based integrated approaches, with clinicians operating as practitioner, partner and leader (Department of Health 2008:9).

For healthcare practitioners, the lesson from Handy (1989) is that change is essential when there are changes in the environment. However, he goes on to argue that change is necessary, if a change in the organization will help it be more successful, even though there are no changes in the environment. In essence then, necessary change can be prompted internally or externally (Handy 1989). As professionals, perioperative practitioners are in a prime position to develop their role and knowledge as lifelong learners. They have a body of professional knowledge that they need to maintain (Illes 2006). Reflective practice is an important tool in facilitating individuals to explore their own practice and examine the clinical decision-making process. It requires individuals to question practice. It is, therefore, important in enabling them to move away from ritualistic practice towards an evidence-based one. This is pertinent in perioperative practice and its development.

Core Topics in Operating Department Practice: Leadership and Management, ed. Brian Smith, Paul Rawling, Paul Wicker and Chris Jones. Published by Cambridge University Press. © Cambridge University Press 2010.

The concept of reflective practice

Reflective practice is defined as 'a set of abilities and skills, to indicate the taking of a critical stance, an orientation to problem solving or state of mind' (Moon 1999:63). This encapsulates the wide range of activities associated with thinking about learning and practice experience. Another view on the process of reflection is that it occurs when an analysis or an evaluation is made of more than one experience and an attempt is made to generalize from that thinking (Cowan 1999). However, Biggs (1999) illustrates the concept of reflection using the example of an image reflected in a mirror being an exact replica of what is in front of it. Set in professional practice, reflection, he argues, gives back not what is but what might be, an improvement on the original. The implication of the notion of improvement is change for the better.

For the purpose of this chapter, reflective practice is perhaps best understood as an approach which promotes autonomous learning that aims to develop a practitioner's understanding and critical thinking skills.

When the descriptor reflective practitioner is used, the usual reference is to adult learners who are engaged in some form of activity, often professional, which they can use to reflect on their strengths, weaknesses and areas for development. They need to be encouraged to use situations, for example group discussions, peer reviews or action learning set meetings, as a basis for reflecting on what they have learned.

Schön (1983) refers to reflective practitioners who are not just skilful or competent but thoughtful, wise and contemplative. He further argues that they are people whose work involves intuition, insight and artistry. Schön (1983) also speaks of the practitioner's draw on intuition in order to do things that feel right. He describes intuition as an emotional response that compliments knowledge and what is already understood about a subject and which enables action to be taken.

The process of reflective practice

Within clinical practice, professionals face unique and challenging situations. They need flexible ways of responding to, and learning from, real situations in order to further their expertise. A tool to facilitate this is reflection. Practical experience is a rich source of learning. However, the experience gained in practice is not enough to maximize the benefit of the experience. Objective analysis is required in order for meaningful learning to occur. The value and importance of reflection in the role of the peri-operative practitioner is that the individual is enabled to develop both personally and professionally. This can result in an evaluation of a situation and subsequent modifying actions as appropriate. Johns (1995) encourages the individual to reflect on how he or she would actually be able to influence a situation. Ghaye & Lillyman (2001) support this in suggesting that it is not enough merely to question things daily, as this will not necessarily lead to improvement. They further argue that one outcome of reflection should be that there are consequences, in that the reflector should come to know the wise, competent and ethical decision to take and have the courage and skills to defend it.

Reflecting on practice should follow a process and be based on a model of reflection. For the purposes of illustrating this point and introducing one model of reflection, the modelling framework of Gibbs (1988) is presented in Fig. 15.1. This model provides a cyclical framework within which the practitioner is facilitated to follow a systematic review of a particular experience through self-questioning. In following the process through, the practitioner ensures that the cycle of reflection is complete and learning is not truncated at an early stage; thus the experience is not wasted.

Stage 1: description

In stage 1, the practitioner recalls the experience and asks the question, 'What actually happened?' The caveat to note here is that early reflection is important as recall is not as accurate after time has

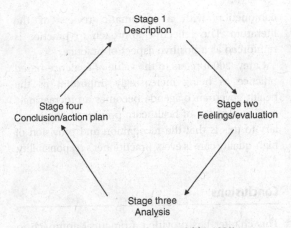

Stage 1
Description

Stage four
Conclusion/action plan

Stage two
Feelings/evaluation

Stage three
Analysis

Figure 15.1. The cycle of reflection (Gibbs 1988).

elapsed. Many people claim to reflect on their practice but take the reflective process no further than this point. If this should happen, the activity has involved remembering the event as opposed to reflecting upon it.

Stage 2: feelings/evaluation

At stage 2 of the process, the practitioner objectively and carefully considers personal feelings at the time, and also an honest consideration of the perceptions of the feelings of other people involved in the experience. Those people are 'significant others', who may be patients, relatives, students, peers or colleagues.

Stage 3: analysis

Here the practitioner starts to make sense of the experience and considers the responses and behaviours that the experience generated. If the experience involved dealing with a distressful or stressful event, it may have justified the inclusion of some non-verbal communication, for example touch. In learning through reflection, the practitioner may want to justify the appropriateness of this action. Benner (1984) identifies touch and person-to-person contact as an example of expert (nursing) practice. At the stage of analysing an experience, the practitioner may be directed to the

literature for further learning support. To this end the theory–practice gap may be reduced. When reflecting on practice with a student or in a clinical supervision setting, the process of analysis plays a significant role.

Stage 4: conclusion/action plan

This is the final stage of the cycle where the practitioner draws the experience to a close. The conclusion is fundamental to the development of an action plan to further the learning or to reflect on the success of the event and to reinforce what action would be taken should a similar experience occur in the future. At this juncture, it may also be useful to revisit the description of the experience again. The cyclical nature of this framework ensures that reflection is ongoing and features as part of the total context of practice and is not a discrete or a one-off activity.

The use of critical incidents as a basis for reflection

The term critical incident comes from history where it refers to some event or situation that marks a significant turning-point or change in the life of a person or institution (Tripp 1993). He gives as examples 'a political party in some social phenomenon (including industrialization, a war or some legal negotiations)'. He goes on to say that 'being major events, this kind of critical incident occurs so rarely in a teacher's lifetime that it alone could not constitute an adequate basis for a professional research file'. While Tripp's work is set in the environment of formal education, there is significant applicability to healthcare practice.

Critical incident analysis is one tool used in the development of nursing practice. Critical incidents are those events that occur in practice which have a significant relevance for those experiencing them. They can be positive or negative in the eyes of the practitioner. Critical incident analysis through the adoption of reflective practice can be effective in improving the healthcare that is provided. Palmer *et al.* (1994) argue that the best possible environment for innovative practice is one where colleagues are not only committed to professional practice but also committed to becoming reflective practitioners.

These writers assert that some might think reflecting on an incident serves to highlight where things have gone wrong, but it actually prevents the practitioner becoming complacent with everyday aspects of work and allowing their practice to become habitual (Palmer *et al.* 1994).

Evidence-based practice and reflection

Evidence-based practice is essential in all contemporary healthcare provision. It is fundamental to effective use of resources and to quality in the outcomes of care delivery. In the move towards evidence-based practice, there needs to be a fundamental willingness for practitioners to examine and analyse their own clinical practice. Reflective practice aids this process (Freshwater 1998).

Given the overriding dominance of the medical profession in healthcare delivery, it is unsurprising that other healthcare practitioners have failed to examine the wider research evidence within care provision (Carey 2000). While this assertion is made in the context of nursing practice, it could be argued that it is pertinent in other clinical fields. Kitson *et al.* (1996) cited by Carey 2000) highlighted that only a small number of healthcare interventions are based on available evidence. Further, Kitson *et al.* (1996) argue that the failure to implement research findings is a result of the imposition of guidelines that are not meaningful to the practitioner, failure to understand standard setting methodologies and failure to examine the implementation from a contextual perspective (Carey 2000). They argue that practice is best developed through an inductive approach. This facilitates creativity, innovation and reflective practice in

conjunction with a systematic review of the literature. The reflective approach to practice is reinforced as a positive aspect of practice.

Carey (2000) refers to the value of evidence-based practice as being increasingly important as the health governance agenda becomes an increasingly explicit element of healthcare provision. The corollary to this is that the recognition and provision of high-quality care is every practitioner's responsibility.

Conclusions

This chapter has provided a practical approach to reflective practice and a stimulus for further exploration of the theories that underpin the activity of reflection. The introduction of the concept of reflection was intended to provide a taster and a foundation for further reading. The literature on reflection is rich and some of this has been drawn upon to illustrate the basic key points here. The intention is to guide the student or practitioner who wishes to embark on the personal development of reflection, and to introduce reflection into their respective practice.

One modelling framework (Gibbs 1988), from many others, has been used to highlight the systematic nature of reflection as a process within personal and professional development in a working environment that requires all healthcare professionals to engage in lifelong learning.

The importance of reflection as a fundamental component of evidence-based practice and its implementation has been outlined. This gave a rationale for the use of reflection and illustrated its role in the provision of quality healthcare.

REFERENCES

Benner, P. (1984). *From Novice to Expert: Excellence and Power in Clinical Nursing Practice*. San Francisco, CA: Addison-Wesley.

Biggs, J. (1999). *Teaching for Quality Learning at University*. Milton Keynes, UK: Open University Press for the Society for Research into Higher Education.

Carey, L. (2000). *Practice Nursing*. London: Baillière Tindall.

Cowan, J. (1999). *On Becoming an Innovative University Teacher*. Milton Keynes, UK: Open University Press for the Society for Research into Higher Education.

Department of Health (1997). *The New NHS: Modern, Dependable*. London: The Stationery Office.

Department of Health (2000). *The NHS Plan: A Plan for Investment, a Plan for Reform*. London: The Stationery Office.

Department of Health (2008). *High Quality Care for All: NHS Next Stage Review Final Report*. London: The Stationery Office.

Freshwater, D. (1998). *Transforming Nursing through Reflective Practice*. Oxford: Blackwell Science.

Ghaye, T. & Lillyman, S. (2001). *Learning Journals and Critical Incidents: Reflective Practice for Health Care Professionals*. London: Quay Books.

Gibbs, G. (1988). *Learning by Doing: A Guide to Teaching and Learning Methods*. Oxford: Oxford Polytechnic.

Handy, C. (1989). *The Age of Unreason*. London: Arrow Books.

Illes, V. (2006). *Really Managing Health Care*, 2nd edn. Milton Keynes, UK: Open University Press.

Johns, C. (1995). The value of reflective practice for nursing. *Journal of Clinical Nursing*, **4**, 22–60.

Moon, J.A. (1999). *Reflection in Own and Professional Development: Theory, Practice*. London: Kogan Page.

Palmer, A., Burns, S. & Bulman, C. (1994). *Pushing Back the Boundaries of Professional Experience: Reflective Practice in Nursing*. Oxford: Blackwell Science.

Schön, D.A. (1983). *The Reflective Practitioner*. San Francisco, CA: Jossy-Bass.

Tripp, D. (1993). *Critical Incidents in Teaching: Developing Professional Judgement*. London: Routledge.

16

New ways of working in perioperative practice

Paul Rawling

Key Learning Points
- Recognize the need for evidence-based practice in perioperative care
- Understand how clinical governance can improve the quality of patient care
- Examine the role of clinical risk management on practice and quality improvement
- Recognize what innovation is and how it can help in delivering efficient patient care

Introduction

Quality in the NHS is viewed as a major issue, borne out by the NHS executive document *Clinical Governance: Quality in the New NHS* (Department of Health 1999a). This raises the question as to why Trusts are apparently not working very quickly towards achieving the aims set out in this document. Is the question 'What do you perceive to be your Trust's "quality improvement strategy"?' a source of mirth in operating departments? Some colleagues may well suggest that none of the three words quality, improvement and strategy should actually be used singly within the workplace let alone together in one sentence. It is a little disappointing that operating departments, and disconcerting for operating department managers, if this reaction takes place. This chapter will question how quality can be improved in operating departments when the management is perceived to be

constrained by cost; it will do so by exploring innovation. It must also be considered how patients perceive the care they receive (Hewison 2004). Care may be delivered in a technically excellent manner but the patients' overall consideration of the quality of care received can sometimes be clouded by the overlong wait for an episode of treatment.

So what is innovation? To the majority of people it means simply something new, an idea, perhaps even something creative. This is essentially true and is relevant to all practice in the healthcare environment. How else will practice progress and patient care develop? It is also apparent that innovation is limited only by our own imagination and the boundaries that we as professionals subconsciously construct around the tasks carried out every day. This chapter aims to demonstrate how practice is changing; roles are remaining the same although other grades of personnel may be capable of carrying out those tasks in a safe and efficient manner.

Efficiency and effectiveness in the operating department

Following the publication of *A Health Service of all the Talents* (Department of Health 2000a), healthcare leaders and managers recognized the need to maximize the contribution to patient care by all the

Core Topics in Operating Department Practice: Leadership and Management, ed. Brian Smith, Paul Rawling, Paul Wicker and Chris Jones. Published by Cambridge University Press. © Cambridge University Press 2010.

staff, in an effective and cost-efficient manner. Bleakley *et al.* (2004) suggest that stress and fatigue among staff are inevitable in a high-pressure, high-risk environment such as the operating department, where organizational targets are set and must be met. Pressure of this nature may be caused by increased turnover of staff, increased sickness levels and incivility and friction within teams.

In 1989 the National Health Service Management Executive VFM Unit published a report entitled *The Management and Utilization of Operating Departments* also known as the Bevan Report. This report suggested that the shortfall of operating department assistants had reached almost 25%. Since this time, has anything changed in the perioperative environment? The report did not compensate for the shortage of trained nursing staff at that time but it did identify a high turnover within this group and difficulties with recruitment and retention. In 2002, Moore suggested that within five years operating departments nationwide could potentially lose up to 25% of skilled registered workers through natural wastage, including retirement, ill health and staff leaving the NHS. Within this study, almost two thirds of operating department managers interviewed stated that they had difficulty recruiting staff of all grades with appropriate skills, a situation which appears to be continuing in 2008.

The changing workforce programme established by the Modernisation Agency (2001) to explore new ways of improving patient care, maximizing staff skills and targeting staff shortages appears largely ineffective at present. Further anecdotal evidence already exists suggesting that support worker roles are being replaced in many Trusts by assistant practitioners. An increasing number of higher education institutions are providing the theoretical learning required by this group in the form of foundation degrees aimed at support workers from various clinical areas including the operating department.

The majority of Trusts have now employed a clinical risk manager and some have gone as far as creating clinical risk departments; these have been chosen, employed and given the remit to champion clinical governance in the clinical environment.

There is a requirement for champions and leaders in every organization and in every department to instil passion, provide explanations and guidance, listen to opinions and, above all, make things happen (House 1996). The author's personal experience has shown that there is a lack of willingness among clinical staff to embrace the overall philosophy of clinical governance. Awareness is increasing as to why everyone within healthcare needs to be involved, to ensure the local delivery of the complex, yet key principles of clinical governance. The question remains as to how clinical governance has affected quality improvement in operating departments.

Cost culture

Operating department managers are faced with important decisions that must be considered while walking a fiscal tightrope. Examples include cancelling operating sessions when there is a shortage of skilled staff or when and from where new equipment should be procured. Experience would indicate that these are not decisions to be taken without every conceivable option being explored. Managers who are faced with decisions of this nature feel threatened or even blamed within the current culture of NHS organizations. As stated in the document produced by the Department of Health (1999a), clinical governance is about culture change within the organization in a systematic and demonstrable way. It is the intention of all managers and senior staff to encourage colleagues to stop ritualistic practices and underpin their practice with good quality evidence. The statement that 'we have always done it this way' is no longer acceptable, although Wicker (1999) believes that in certain circumstances this approach might deliver at least a standard of care that could be considered minimal. It has become everyone's duty to implement evidence-based practice into everyday use, as stated in *A First Class Service* (Department of Health 1998). Hutchins (1992) suggests that the way forward is to empower people and give them the opportunity to tackle the problems identified, providing them with the skills to resolve these problems and issues. This is not always the experience in all operating departments. It could be suggested that sometimes operating department managers do not feel that they can devolve any part of their overall control to employees, even though this is part of leadership and culture change (Donaldson & Muir-Gray 1998). The issues of most concern in operating departments appear to be conceptualized in cost, which is the key item on the management agenda, and this is supported by Donaldson & Muir-Gray (1998).

Expanding roles in perioperative care

Registered nurses and operating department practitioners (ODP) now undertake a broader range of roles including ones that were traditionally carried out by medical staff, such as non-medical anaesthetists, critical care practitioners (physician assistants), surgical care practitioners (non-physician surgeons), first assistants and emergency care practitioners. A clear need is being demonstrated for flexible working within the workforce. This has been discussed by Stokes & Warden (2004) as leaving a basic care gap, which could potentially be filled by support workers.

Should professional staff continue to be protective of their roles or should they broaden their view and examine the overall efficiency of the model of care they currently use and support? Current service provision drives operating department and hospital managers inexorably toward developing all staff groups into roles that may be potentially difficult to fill. This may be stimulated by several factors, such as the European Working Time Directive, a reduction in medical staff numbers and a reduction in the number of nurses or ODPs wishing to undertake a career in a particular area such as the operating theatre. It must be borne in mind that current numbers of professional staff being

produced by higher education institutions may not currently match the clinical need.

Purdy & Banks (2001) comment on society's expectations of healthcare services and support the notion that the general public wishes to be treated in a safe and consistent manner at a time when it is required, with little or no evidence to suggest that the public feels that the care should be provided by a specific professional group.

> **Reflective point**
>
> - What is your perception of the requirement to improve the effectiveness of the current service model employed in your department?

Many ideas and policies have emerged in recent years intended to ensure that the services provided by the NHS are delivered with the needs of patients in mind. These ideas and policies are of great potential value but their implications for professional roles and the organization of the NHS has not yet been fully appreciated.

The Department of Health document *The New NHS: Modern, Dependable* (1997) highlights political support for innovation of this nature in a move toward greater efficiency, value for money and twenty-first century care for patients at a time and place to best suit the patient, who is the end user of the service. Quite clearly, partnerships across NHS, professional bodies and higher education institutions and professional groups working in a culture of openness and cooperation, as suggested by (Howkins & Thornton 2002), will be required for success, if indeed progress is actually what all desire. This belief is supported by Muir-Gray (2001), who comments on the need for acceleration of change within clinical practice. The document *Human Resources in The NHS Plan* (Department of Health 2002) focuses on changing the way staff work, for the benefit of the patients, and calls for more staff working differently, with investment and reform to enable NHS staff to take forward *The NHS Plan* (Department of Health 2000a). Innovation of this nature is designed to optimize the workload of professional staff, allowing them to undertake duties commensurate with their knowledge and skills.

The role of non-registered staff groups

The government's assertion that lifelong learning is aimed at providing all staff groups with the ability to update knowledge and skills to ensure provision of high-quality effective care (Department of Health 1998) applies equally to registered and non-registered staff groups. It is conservatively estimated that approximately 100 000 support workers are employed in the UK under as many as 300 different titles and a range of roles (Spilsbury & Meyer 2004). Learning is seen as key to a better future for individual staff and the NHS itself (Department of Health 1998, Wilkinson *et al.* 2004). It is becoming more apparent that it is necessary to enhance the scope of practice of skilled but unregistered staff to fill the skill's gap that is emerging as professional roles continue to develop and change.

The formalization of support worker training has been evident in the increased use of National Vocational Qualification (NVQ) levels 2 and 3 within operating departments over recent years. The NVQ level 3 was the former entry level qualification for the ODP. It has now evolved to become a diploma of higher education and will eventually become a degree level entry profession. Role expansion for support workers is, therefore, a natural progression provided that the role of the support worker is accurately defined and formal theoretical education and training is developed and applied nationally. It should be remembered that nursing staff are not currently obliged to possess a specific perioperative qualification to carry out that role; however, they must have appropriate training and maintain competence within their scope of practice.

The use of support workers could be advocated as one method of overcoming continuous staff shortages within certain clinical areas (Chang 1995,

Spilsbury & Meyer 2004), which certainly includes operating departments. Little published literature or empirical data are available surrounding the issue of operating department support workers and their roles, although a number of discussion papers are available regarding the scrub role. However, literature does exist in relation to support workers in other areas of clinical practice. The papers attempt to define the perceived demarcation of nursing and non-nursing roles as being fluid or blurred. The crossing of occupational boundaries has been suggested to be an essential element of delivering high-quality care (Department of Health 2001a) and that workforce planning must be based on competencies required to deliver services (Masterson 2002). It could be suggested that much of the work carried out by qualified practitioners of all disciplines within operating departments is duplicated in much of the support workers' current roles. The literature suggests that very few healthcare tasks and procedures are legally restricted to any one professional group or even the professions (Masterson 2002). Restrictions appear only to exist through organizational and professional custom and practice. Timmons & Tanner (2004) and Spilsbury & Meyer (2004) confirm that role boundaries between professional groups and support workers are becoming blurred in the operating department, which is technically, though not professionally, correct. Allen (2001) considers boundaries between the roles of professional and support workers and suggests that these boundaries are not fixed by statute but are essentially a social construct of professional staff based on deep-seated professional protectionism of current roles without consideration of how current roles have evolved. It is clear that the overlapping roles of operating department staff, in relation to the economics of staff shortage and increasing skill levels, indicate a need to explore staffing options. *Agenda for Change* (Department of Health 2004) demonstrates a clear intention to allow support workers to develop and to undertake tasks currently carried out by professional staff.

The majority of publications on this topic have been written by nurses and demonstrate some degree of bias regarding ownership of roles. The results focused largely on the accountability of registered staff and the perceived fact that non-registered support workers are not accountable. The fact that non-registered support workers are not professionally accountable does not mean that they are not accountable in law (Dimond 2002) or to their employers or the patients themselves, which appeared to be the belief of some of the registered respondents. It is recognized that the non-registered workers undertake a large and diverse range of tasks that contain specific skills, and it was also recognized that experiential learning and self-teaching amongst this group of staff challenge some of the preconceived ideas about competency held by some professional staff. Employers have a legal obligation to ensure that all staff are 'fit for purpose' in that they can carry out the tasks they are undertaking, with clear emphasis placed on patient safety.

The data in publications support the beliefs of the staff group that the actors within the research came from, either professional or non-registered groups. Conclusions were again supportive of the registered staff groups views and beliefs and at times focused on the history of nursing and other related professions and not on the future of healthcare as the government of the day or patients may wish to see it.

The joint statements of the Perioperative Care Collaborative (2004a, 2004b) support the view that national occupational standards should be available for support workers in the operating department through the NVQ framework or an equivalent nationally recognized award, along with guidelines for role definition. The statements acknowledge that some Trusts have implemented competency-based programmes, many with links to the NHS *Knowledge and Skills Framework* and with policies to support role development of support workers.

The greatest problem within the issue of support workers in the operating department is that of role definition. The roles undertaken by support workers vary across the country so much that clearly defining roles would be extremely difficult.

However, evidence suggests that the time of professional staff was freed up as a consequence of the appropriate use of support workers (Ormandy *et al.* 2004) and that increasing the skills of support workers did not de-skill professional staff.

The use of support workers in a scrub role was discussed in the Bevan Report (National Health Service Management Executive VFM Unit 1989) and even then caused consternation amongst the registered members of staff. It should be remembered that ODPs were not statutorily registered until October 2004 and may have been viewed in a similar light. Chang *et al.* (2005) imply that registered staff may be substituted for non-registered staff as a cost-saving initiative, which may potentially be true in some Trusts. Delegation and supervision of support workers is fundamental to the role, but from experience does not consistently happen in the clinical area owing, in part, to poor staffing levels (Stokes & Warden 2004), thus indicating non-fulfilment of the professional role. Professionally registered practitioners must be aware that the perioperative workforce of the future is potentially going to develop in ways that are out of line with traditional health professional roles and their perception of how perioperative care should be shaped. These factors not only enhance the need for robust regulatory systems but may challenge existing unidisciplinary regulatory arrangements.

Staff shortages and skill mix

A study by Ormandy *et al.* (2004) shows that healthcare support workers within critical care environments are a valuable and effective resource, which should be good news for hard-pressed operating department managers and cash-deficient Trusts. In this study, perceptions of key actors were sought using questionnaires, interviews, focus groups and non-participant observation over a number of sites. All respondents were nurses, which potentially could have introduced bias as further staff groups may have had an interest. The findings suggested that role definition for support workers was problematic in that agreement amongst nurses across sites and within units could not be achieved. The overall outcome of the research was that almost 80% of respondents believed they had more time for key tasks. A list of tasks deemed suitable for support workers was drawn up and agreed, illustrating the need for clinical staff involvement in role development and training for support workers. The key to enhancing the role of the operating department support workers and maintaining patient safety is clarity of role definition. Validated formal structured education on a national level, as discussed by McKenna *et al.* (2004), focuses on the reduction of ad hoc roles and the improvement of professional staff skills in appropriate delegation of tasks and in acceptance of responsibility and accountability. Statutory regulation of support workers would be advantageous in the implementation of this innovation. Ward & Wood (2000) suggest that implicit relevance of training must be demonstrated to increase motivation of learners and ensure fitness for purpose and patient safety.

In a climate of cost saving, equipping professional staff with perioperative skills is also becoming more difficult in terms of maintaining the current level of service. The alleviation of staff shortages and improved efficiency and cost-effectiveness must be considered (Chang 1995). A cost saving could be achieved if turnover of staff was reduced, and morale may be improved at the same time as this would relieve some of the pressure on the professional staff. Key government papers identify that Trusts are required to deliver consistent and high-quality care to patients (Department of Health 1997, 1998, 1999b, 2000b). To achieve the required objectives, each Trust must maintain a workforce capable of meeting the changing needs within healthcare. The changes the NHS is experiencing are rapid and unsettling for all staff.

It is clear that overlapping roles of operating department staff in relation to the economics of staff shortage and increasing skill levels needs further exploration. Innovations that fit with current organizational skill mix, values and norms have a greater chance of success and would be aided by interventions aimed at reducing the impact of environmental stressors such as workload and staffing. This should go some way to improve staff retention, as suggested by Chang *et al.* (2005).

The role of innovation

The supporters of the suggested innovation concerning use of support workers are multidisciplinary, are keen to support change and are growing in number. This is evidenced by the increasing number of clinical areas that are currently utilizing or developing the support worker grade. They appear to believe in *The NHS Plan* (Department of Health 2002; Chapter 2: *More Staff Working Differently*) to meet demand for services and the creation of a more flexible workforce. Most perioperative practitioners of all disciplines are (or at least should be) acutely aware of current deficiencies in staffing recruitment and retention within operating departments. Change agents, operating department trainers and managers, do appear interested in the development of the support worker group of staff.

Change management and leadership

Innovation leads to the need for a change strategy and requires reducing resistance to the innovation that is caused by fear and uncertainty (Copnell 1998). A clear vision that the change is of value to the stakeholders is paramount and must be communicated well in an honest, open and transparent manner, as suggested by Moullin (2002), along with clarifying for staff, users and partners the direction that the organization must take to achieve the desired state. A shared decision-making process involving the groups of individuals who will be directly affected needs to be put in place through the use of focus and steering groups and the use of a transformational leadership style (Mullins 1999). It is important that all stakeholders are involved and are empowered through a decentralized approach (Scott & Caress 2005). The model proposed by Protchaska & DiClementi (1982) for organizational change is based on the concept of balance in that change occurs when there are more motivational forces in favour of change than those favouring the status quo (Howarth & Morrison 2000). In the context of this chapter, current clinical areas reflect this. Therefore, it will be vital to engage all stakeholders and motivate them in favour of the change, if possible at an early stage. Additionally, it has been suggested by Upton & Brooks (1995) that some rapid change is necessary to enhance the motivation of the stakeholders. Where subordinate acceptance is crucial but conflict still possible, the preferred leadership style adopted will be participative, and group involvement is the way to achieve engagement toward change where fundamental changes to structure or practice are required.

Strong leadership both formal and informal will be required, as will the creation of a climate in which participants feel free to communicate without threat. It is important to create a culture of trust and not control, which is supported by Braganza & Ward (2001), who favour incremental change and suggest that people are often at the centre of failings in strategic innovations. Howkins & Thornton (2002) emphasize the need for cooperation when managing and leading innovation. However, it is inevitable that conflict will occur; this is partly a consequence of human nature as all tend to feel threatened by change that they are not fully involved in and perhaps do not feel necessary. Conflict need not be looked upon as negative, however, but can be viewed as positive and useful, and may actually be inevitable in organizations where groups of individuals with differing views and ideas coexist, as in the multiprofessional team.

Human nature will not allow individuals to accept change outright, but rather prompts a need to question why what is being done now needs to be changed. Adams (1996) suggests that the reasoning behind this view is that 'change adds new information to the universe, information that we don't know. Our knowledge – as a percentage of all things that can be known – goes down a tick every time something changes.' Evidence is out there and Muir-Gray (1997:67) states that we must 'use it or lose it'. It remains the author's belief that people who find, appraise and use evidence contribute to changing the culture of the organization in which they work.

Patient and staff safety is vital in the twenty-first century: the technology, skills and knowledge are available and, under clinical governance guidelines, can be used within all NHS Trusts. Handy (1995) and Hussey (2000) have differing views but agree that change of any kind can actually be comfortable when incremental, and this can also be applied to culture change within organizations. Clinical governance and quality improvement in the NHS continues at a pace and has never been comfortable for front-line staff, but Hussey (2000) suggests that it is important to retain loyalty and maintain positive motivation of the people (practitioners) affected. This can be seen in the operating department employees, who on occasion appear demoralized and unmotivated, possibly because of the pressure of work and the personal and professional pressures inherent with continuous change.

A whole system approach to quality improvement across boundaries, including a robust arrangement for identifying and remedying risks and poor performance, is required to progress perioperative care. Dissemination of information is often lacking, as is the leadership to ensure changes to process and culture are implemented. To improve quality standards requires knowledge of the complex nature of quality and all its facets. Bone & Griggs (1989:36) suggest that the intangible basics of quality are 'commitment, competence and communication'; as organizations' quality standards are based on policies and goals, employees need to know what these are. Trust management commitment must be transferred to everyone within the organization.

Secker-Walker & Merrit (1997) consider that good communication with patients is an effective means of preventing litigation when they perceive something has gone wrong. The author believes that organizational communication with the staff to ensure awareness of clinical governance and its role in quality improvement within the organization is at least equally as important. Other chapters in this volume expand on change management and leadership.

Risk assessment

Operating departments have made progress in risk management over recent years. The incidence of critical incident reporting has quadrupled and Secker-Walker & Merrit (1997) suggest that this is fundamental to the management of the clinical risk process. The communication of feedback from incident reporting is potentially too slow to maintain momentum and clinical staff motivation. Operating departments present special problems in relation to clinical risk as patients in this part of the organization's care process are potentially at their most vulnerable, particularly when anaesthetized and undergoing surgery, and their safety is left entirely to the staff in the department. Despite organizations being keen to engage with clinical risk assessment, Neal (1998) suggests that employers embarking on clinical risk programmes do not utilize their workforce to their advantage. Clinical risk management strategies are an effective method of involving employees in quality improvement and allow staff a sense of personal ownership of quality improvement (Fox 1991). Risk management means maximizing resources for patient care, controlling or minimizing risk to all users of Trust premises, controlling or eliminating risks that may have adverse effects on quality of care, and maintaining health, safety and welfare of staff. It must be stated that staff within departments are the most crucial resource available to all managers.

Evidence-based practice and quality issues

A registered practitioner becomes accountable through the professional standards or codes of conduct of the particular discipline, which require maintenance of the currency of knowledge and practice in line with the requirement for continuous professional development. As research continues, evidence becomes more readily available yet is still out of reach of many practitioners. White (1997) suggests that evidence-based practice emphasizes the importance of experimental evidence over practitioner experience, which is considered a weaker form of evidence and arising at least in part from the maintenance of ritualistic practices. Protocols, guidelines, policies and procedures are slowly growing in number and complexity. Managers are possibly now worried because of this, although the situation could also be viewed as a great opportunity for staff to be involved in policy and procedure making; using the latest evidence, gained from systematic reviews, there is now virtually a blank page to start work from.

Muir-Gray (1997) infers that the key components of an evidence-based health service is an organization with the capacity to generate evidence, which operating departments clearly have, and the flexibility to incorporate evidence into practice, through individuals and teams who have the knowledge, ability and training to find, appraise and use research evidence. The Department of Health (1999a) *Clinical Governance* White Paper sets out the main components of quality improvement, which includes the use of evidence-based practice that is supported by the whole organization and implemented into everyday practice. Clinical audit, both nationally and locally, is an effective method of measuring potential improvements in outcomes and in generating evidence. This is a tool that remains underutilized. Audit can guide the progress of quality improvement within practice, which is our overall aim when it is related to caring for our patients.

A number of quality improvement models and ideas exist, most relating to industry but a few are easily transferable to the health service sector. Professional healthcare personnel are traditionally uncomfortable with theories of quality improvement derived from industry because of the perception that clinical outcomes could then be equated to products in industry (Donaldson & Muir-Gray 1998).

Donaldson & Muir-Gray (1998) suggest that all the theories have common threads, including leadership, staff empowerment, teamwork, a strong customer focus and prevention rather than correction of adverse outcomes. These threads can be seen in the perioperative environment but lack the integration required to make the system work effectively. At present, it would appear that quality improvement is failing through weaknesses in staff education, because research evidence is under-valued and because of the corporate division of staff into small groups and cliques.

Clinical audit is almost universally recognized as a method of evaluating the quality of the care provided. Clinical audit is the measuring of the effectiveness of what is currently done against set standards (Berk *et al.* 2003). The recognition of high-quality care provision is equally as important as the recognition of poor practice. The key to clinical audit is the ability to be involved as a practitioner and to embrace any change implementation.

The author's experience suggests that audit has become a 'buzz' word within operating departments. The fact that audit now has a very public profile, with the development of audit departments within Trusts, can help when it comes to the need for practice to be based on evidence and for fulfilling clinical governance strategies and the targets of the NHS Clinical Negligence Scheme for Trusts. Clinical audit guidelines currently suggest that identifying a subject is best done through the trigger of a significant or adverse event within a department. Critical incident reporting has uncovered a number of potential audit subjects in the operating department, including the problems encountered when simply sending for patients.

Essentially, audit allows practitioners to reflect on the service they currently deliver to patients against evidence-based set standards. However few members of staff appear to understand that audit is far from just the collection of numeric data used

to judge staff performance or provide evidence of rising costs. The multiprofessional collaborative nature of clinical audit enables greater versatility within the process of care. It must be noted, however, that clinical audit is not the great panacea that will enable change to be successfully implemented and maintained (Craig & Smyth 2002). Within any department, it should not be considered that all practice is perfect. Clinical audit can be immensely useful in 'areas of guideline related practice' (Craig & Smyth 2002:261) that may be considered deficient and would benefit from remodelling, leading to:

- more appropriate standards: policies/procedures
- increased proficiency of staff: training/development
- early problem recognition: incident reporting
- effective problem solving: risk management
- better care and service: improved patient safety and lower number of complaints
- pride in common achievement: ownership.

The author believes that quality improvement is about discipline, procedures, standards and, in healthcare, culture change and the way staff think. Fox (1991) suggests a total quality management trilogy – quality commitment, quality systems and quality measurement – and this could be considered a realistic way to make quality improvement happen in the operating department. Commitment of a Trust to quality begins with a strategic policy, which is better known as a mission or vision statement. The vast majority of Trusts and departments now have these.

Reflective point

- What are the mission statements of your Trust and department?

Quality systems require involvement of every directorate and department within a Trust. It may be necessary to develop procedures, standards, processes and resources (e.g. *The Essence of Care*; Department of Health 2001a) and move toward the previously used nursing process strategy.

Fox (1991) believes that quality improvement cannot be sustained without the use of evaluation-based measurement techniques (audit). The author feels that the total quality management trilogy of Fox (1991) is workable within the operating department context. It must be underpinned by everyone being involved, and everyone must have a shared responsibility if a patient makes a complaint, amounting to total involvement from the top of the Trust to the bottom.

New concepts and often-complex ideas, theories and models remain difficult to implement. However, without the seniority required for implementation on an organizational stage, practitioners will struggle to improve quality through changing practice. Much of the literature leads to a conclusion that, although many experts extol the virtues of quality improvement programmes, quality improvement is a process lacking the end point suggested by use of the word programme. Quality improvement is a dynamic concept and is ultimately a journey not a destination.

In the perioperative context, Handy's (1995) analogy of the boiling frog describes the beliefs of many perioperative staff members, apart from a few progressive individuals who appear prepared to change their behaviour when faced with discontinuous change. Garbett (1998) sums up current views towards quality improvement when he suggests that no practitioners wish to provide substandard care though this is perhaps what is sometimes provided. Is this substandard care what anyone would wish for if they themselves were the patients.

Conclusions

Quality in certain contexts can be free. This said, in the operating department working as a single practice unit it is potentially possible to provide the wrong care or substandard care when patients are most vulnerable through the current inability to implement evidence. Implementation of a quality improvement programme, the maintenance of a continuous process of improvement and the elimination of barriers to implementation of research evidence are issues to be considered by everyone.

The research evidence available on the subject of non-registered staff roles is plentiful although not specific to perioperative areas. Some operating departments already use this group in enhanced roles previously undertaken by professional staff. The public and these staff members deserve protection from poor practice and litigation, respectively. That protection at the present time is provided through the appropriateness of the task being delegated, the level of supervision provided by individual professional staff members and the robustness of operating department policies and guidelines.

REFERENCES

Adams, S. (1996). *The Dilbert Principle. A Cubicle's Eye View of Bosses, Meetings, Management Fads and Other Workplace Afflictions.* New York: Harper Collins.

Allen, D. (2001). *The Changing Shape of Nursing Practice: The Role of Nurses in the Hospital Division of Labour.* London: Routledge.

Berk, M., Callaly, T. & Hyland, M. (2003). The evolution of clinical audit as a tool for quality improvement. *Journal of Evaluation in Clinical Practice,* 9, 251–257.

Bleakley, A., Hobbs, A., Boyden, J. & Walsh, L. (2004). Safety in operating theatres: improving teamwork through team resource management. *Journal of Workplace Learning,* 16, 2.

Bone, D. & Griggs, R. (1989). *Quality at Work.* London: Kogan Page.

Braganza, A. & Ward, J. (2001). Implementing strategic innovation: supporting people over the design and implementation boundary. *Strategic Change,* 10, 103–113.

Chang, A.M. (1995). Perceived functions and usefulness of health service support workers. *Journal of Advanced Nursing,* 21, 61–74.

Chang, E.M., Hancock, K.M., Johnson, A., Daly, A. & Jackson, D. (2005). Role stress in nurses: review of related factors and strategies for moving forward. *Nursing and Health Sciences,* 7, 57–65.

Copnell, B. (1998). Understanding change in clinical practice. *Nursing Inquiry,* 5, 2–10.

Craig, J.V. & Smyth, R.L. (2002). *The Evidence Based Practice Manual for Nurses*. Edinburgh: Churchill Livingstone.

Department of Health (1997). *The New NHS: Modern, Dependable*. London: The Stationery Office.

Department of Health (1998). *A First Class Service: Quality in the New NHS*. London: The Stationery Office.

Department of Health (1999a). *Clinical Governance: Quality in the New NHS*. London: The Stationery Office.

Department of Health (1999b). *Making a Difference: Strengthening the Nursing, Midwifery and Health Visiting Contribution to Health and Healthcare*. London: The Stationery Office.

Department of Health (2000a). *A Health Service of all the Talents*. London: The Stationery Office.

Department of Health (2000b). *The NHS Plan: A Plan for Investment, a Plan for Reform*. London: The Stationery Office.

Department of Health (2001a). *The Essence of Care*. London: The Stationery Office.

Department of Health (2001b). *Investment and Reform for NHS Staff: Taking Forward the NHS Plan*. London: The Stationery Office.

Department of Health (2002). *Human Resources in the NHS Plan*. Leeds: Human Resource Performance Framework, NHS Executive.

Department of Health (2004). *Agenda for Change*. London: The Stationery Office.

Dimond, B. (2002). *Legal Aspects of Nursing*, 3rd edn. London: Longman.

Donaldson, L.J. & Muir-Gray, J.A. (1998). Clinical governance, a quality duty of care for health organisations. *Quality in Health Care*, **7**, 527–544.

Fox, R. (1991). *Making Quality Happen: Six Steps to Total Quality Management*. Roseville, NJ: McGraw-Hill.

Garbett, R. (1998). Do the right thing. *Nursing Times*, **94**, 28–29.

Handy, C. (1995). *The Age of Unreason*, 2nd edn. London: Arrow.

Hewison, A. (2004). *Management for Nurses and Health Professionals*. Oxford: Blackwell.

House, M. (1996). *Confessions of a Quality Expert: A Systematic Approach to Implementing Total Quality*. Eastham, UK: Tudor Business Publishing.

Howarth, J. & Morrison, T. (2000). Identifying and implementing pathways for organisational change: using the framework for the assessment of children and their families as a case example. *Child and Family Social Work*, **5**, 245–254.

Howkins, E. & Thornton, C. (2002). *Managing and Leading Innovation in Health Care*. London: Baillière Tindall.

Hussey, D.E. (2000). *How to Manage Organisational Change*, 2nd edn. London: Kogan Page.

Hutchins, D. (1992). *Achieve Total Quality*. London: Fitzwilliam.

Masterson, A. (2002). Cross boundary working: a macro political analysis of the impact on professional roles. *Journal of Clinical Nursing*, **11**, 331–339.

McKenna, H.P., Hasson, F. & Keeney, S. (2004). Patient safety and quality of care: the role of the health care assistant. *Journal of Nursing Management*, **12**, 452–459.

Modernisation Agency (2001). *Changing Workforce Programme*. London: The Stationery Office.

Moore, S. (2002). The staffing of the operating theatre: how far have we come since Bevan? *Technic*, **221**, 16–19.

Moullin, M. (2002). *Delivering Excellence in Health and Social Care*. Milton Keynes, UK: Open University Press.

Muir-Gray, J.A. (1997). *Evidence Based Healthcare: How to Make Health Policy and Management Decisions*. Edinburgh: Churchill Livingstone.

Muir-Gray, J.A. (2001). *Evidence Based Healthcare: How to Make Health Policy and Management Decisions*, 2nd edn. Edinburgh: Churchill Livingstone.

Mullins, L. (1999). *Management and Organisational Behaviour*. London: Pitman.

NHS Management Executive VFM Unit (1989). *Staffing and Utilisation of Operating Theatres: A Study Conducted Under the Guidance of a Steering Group [Bevan Report]*. Leeds: NHS Management Executive VFM Unit.

Neal, K. (1998). A framework for managing risk. *Nursing Times Learning Curve*, **1**, 4–5.

Ormandy, P., Long, A., Hulme, C.T. & Johnson, M. (2004). The role of the senior healthcare worker in critical care. *Nursing in Critical Care*, **9**, 151–158.

Perioperative Care Collaborative (2004a). *Delegation: The Support Worker in the Scrub Role. Position Statement*. London: Perioperative Care Collaborative.

Perioperative Care Collaborative (2004b). *Optimising the Contribution of the Perioperative Support Worker. Position Statement*. London: Perioperative Care Collaborative.

Protchaska, J. & DiClementi, C. (1982). Trans-theoretical therapy: towards a more integrative model of change. *Psychotherapy: Theory, Research and Practice*, **19**, 276–288.

Purdy, M. & Banks, D. (2001). *The Sociology and Politics of Health. A Reader*. London: Routledge.

Scott, L. & Caress, A. (2005). Shared governance and shared leadership: meeting the challenges of implementation. *Journal of Nursing Management*, **13**, 4–12.

Secker-Walker, J. & Merrit, H. (1997). Risk in clinical care. *Journal of Nursing Management*, **3**, 22–23.

Spilsbury, K. & Meyer, J. (2004). Use, misuse and non-use of health care assistants: understanding the use of health care assistants in a hospital setting. *Journal of Nursing Management*, **12**, 411–418.

Stokes, J. & Warden, A. (2004). The changing role of the healthcare assistant. *Nursing Standard*, **7**, 51.

Timmons, S. & Tanner, J. (2004). A disputed occupational boundary: operating theatre nurses and operating department practitioners. *Sociology of Health and Illness*, **26**, 645–666.

Upton, T. & Brooks, B. (1995). *Managing Change in the NHS*. London: Kogan Page.

Ward, J. & Wood, C. (2000). Education and training of healthcare staff: barriers to its success. *European Journal of Cancer Care*, **9**, 80–85.

White, S.J. (1997). Evidence based practice and nursing: the new panacea? *British Journal of Nursing*, **6**, 175–178.

Wicker, P. (1999). Editorial comment. *British Journal of Theatre Nursing*, **1**, 24–25.

Wilkinson, J.E., Rushmer, R.K. & Davies, H.T.O. (2004). Clinical governance and the learning organisation. *Journal of Nursing Management*, **12**, 105–113.

17

Damned if you do and damned if you don't: whistle blowing in perioperative practice

Chris Jones

Key Learning Points

- Understand the moral aspects of whistle blowing
- Identify the consequences of whistle blowing

Introduction

There can be few perioperative practitioners who do not prefer the work of some surgeons to that of others. Some surgeons make the work look easy. They are calm under pressure. They use the minimum amount of equipment. Other surgeons just seem to have 'an unusual amount of bad luck'. But for the operating department practitioner or nurse who witnesses this phenomenon, there will be a question that will occur again and again: 'How much poor practice could I stand to watch before I spoke out and said something?'

Dilemmas over what should be spoken about in public and the best way to communicate dissatisfaction with standards at work are deep and complex. At one extreme, simply voicing concerns at work will be enough to rectify an unfortunate situation. At the other extreme, no amount of 'going through the appropriate channels' will be enough to correct even gross lapses in standards. In these circumstances, the employee has to face the prospect of drawing attention to the situation in the most difficult way possible, by whistle blowing (Shah 2005).

In this chapter the moral aspects of whistle blowing will be foremost in the discussion. The changes in legislation surrounding whistle blowing since the mid 1990s will enter the discussion where they are relevant. The main focus of the discussion will be on the moral repercussions of whistle blowing.

Whistle blowing has a long tradition and everybody involved in perioperative care will be able to think of famous cases that have been the subject of press reports. Numerous official reports have pointed to a culture of secrecy in operating departments that has permitted a code of silence to develop (McColgan 2000). For example, Julia Hartley Brewer reported in the *Guardian* in 2000 that 'The disgraced gynaecologist, Rodney Ledward, was able to severely maim hundreds of women patients because of a hospital culture in which consultants were treated as "gods" and junior staff were afraid of "telling tales", the official inquiry into his conduct reported yesterday.' Mr Ledward botched hundreds of operations during his 16 years at the William Harvey Hospital in Ashford, Kent because he was protected by a combination of 'failures in senior NHS management', the 'old boy network' and a 'climate of fear and retribution', which prevented colleagues from reporting their concerns about his surgical skills.

This is by no means an isolated case. Poor practice has been allowed to flourish in the past because of a pervasive climate of fear in which members of staff were afraid to speak out and blow the whistle.

Core Topics in Operating Department Practice: Leadership and Management, ed. Brian Smith, Paul Rawling, Paul Wicker and Chris Jones. Published by Cambridge University Press. © Cambridge University Press 2010.

Table 17.1 Examples of problems and actions

Problem	Reported to
A senior house officer is persistently rude to patients	Operating department manager
A student nurse is persistently late	The university faculty of health
There is a repeated lack of intensive care beds	The Health Care Commission
Ingrained racist attitudes among staff	The local newspaper
A surgeon seems to have a higher than expected patient mortality	The General Medical Council

What is whistle blowing?

It is not entirely clear what constitutes whistle blowing (Firtko & Jackson 2005). At its most simple level, it might mean 'the reporting of poor standards in order to improve the situation'. This might mean letting the manager know what is on your mind in order that your problem can be rectified (Shah 2005). Arguably, however, this is not what most people would regard as whistle blowing. In many respects, what counts as whistle blowing is difficult to define. In Table 17.1, what would constitute whistle blowing and why would it be called such a name? The simple act of reporting something unsatisfactory is not enough to make it whistle blowing. There has to be other aspects to an act of 'reporting' to make it whistle blowing. But what are those other aspects? And how does the individual's duty to improve a situation balance with other responsibilities that they may have to colleagues, the employer and themselves.

Does whistle blowing imply going outside of the organization?

From the evidence of many years of classroom discussions with perioperative practitioners, there seems to be little sympathy for the view that simple reporting is enough to constitute whistle blowing. Genuine whistle blowing implies in some respect going outside of the organization for redress. The staff member has had no luck going through the internal channels and has had to resort to taking the fight beyond the walls of the operating room. The staff member has attempted to rectify the situation by bringing outside pressure to bear on the situation. This, in itself, requires some courage (Shah 2005). Nobody wants to be the 'snitch'. However, the goal is a worthy one: to improve the standard of performance in the operating department.

An obvious first question here is how far away from the walls of the operating department does somebody have to be to be considered outside. Operating departments are closed and intimate communities. Their members share dramatic and often disturbing events. Even practitioners from other operating rooms within the same Trust can seem like outsiders. Does 'going through the channels' in an operating room mean taking the problem as far as the operating department manager, and no further? Would, for instance, taking the problem of the rude senior house officer in Table 17.1 beyond the operating department manager to someone higher up in the Trust constitute whistle blowing? Such a person would be an employee of the same organization after all, even if they were not part of the same actual team. What is more, the Trust member would be bound by the same duty to maintain confidentiality as all other parties.

Where are professional bodies situated in terms of being 'inside' or 'outside'? Would reporting unacceptable behaviour or standards directly to the Nursing and Midwifery Council or the General Medical Council (GMC) constitute going outside of the organization? These bodies are charged with the responsibility of protecting standards of professional practice for the public. It is hard to imagine how they might be regarded as being outside of normal channels. Indeed, each time a scandal breaks regarding medical malfeasance, the allegation is heard that the GMC in particular is too close to the medical professionals it is supposed to be policing.

It is easier to see how reporting concerns to a member of parliament (MP) might be considered going outside normal structures. Certainly it is an MP's job to be aware of problems in as sensitive an area as hospital care. Perhaps if matters relating to public policy are raised by the events that are worrying the staff member, the MP might be an appropriate person to report concerns to. However, it is also the case that the MP might bring to the situation a set of priorities other than improving the state of affairs in your operating department. The MP is, after all, a politician with a range of political objectives to push forward beyond that of improving the health service. This other set of priorities might turn a genuine problem into a political football, which ends far away from where the initiator intended.

If there are difficulties with reporting problems to an MP, these are amplified when considering the prospect of involving the press. A journalist might have little regard for the improvements that an individual would like to see in their unit and may see no further than filling space in today's paper. That said, some of the most telling acts of whistle blowing have involved the press. The notable case of Graham Pink, whose disquiet was expressed through the pages of the *Guardian* is a graphic example of this sort (Freedom to Care 2008).

In order to assist in deciding who to alert concerning poor practice, a list of 'prescribed persons' has been developed and added as an appendix to the Pubic Interest Disclosure Act in 2003. This appendix lists the special interest of various individuals and organizations who might be turned to when a staff member feels that their concerns are being ignored. This might include the Food Standards Agency, the Serious Fraud Office or the Health and Safety Executive.

A list of these 'prescribed persons' is usually included as part of an NHS Trust's whistle blowing policy. It is common practice for operating departments to have ready access to these Trust policies, on paper and online. In addition to this, the Trust might nominate a person or persons to act as the point of initial contact for worried members of staff.

As reasonable as it might seem to appoint an internal 'first response' officer, it is not clear that these safeguards would have helped in some of the most high-profile whistle blowing cases in the NHS. In the case of Graham Pink and in the case of Steven Bolsin, who brought to light the poor mortality figures from the Bristol children's cardiac surgical service in 1995, senior management were quite aware of the initial doubts and concerns. In both cases, the internal channels had been well appraised of these doubts. In both cases, it was the involvement of outside agencies that turned a local dispute into a cause célèbre. In the case of Bristol, a senior manager was disciplined for his role in the dispute.

Does whistle blowing imply a breach of confidentiality?

At one level, it seems obvious that whistle blowing must imply a breach of confidentiality (Firtko & Jackson 2005). Most people observe events every day which they do not regard as ideal. But with some of those events the choice is made to keep it within the family, so to speak. The world would be intolerable if everyone reported every transgression they observed. Yet it is precisely this wish to avoid the 'stool pigeon' role that allows bad, unethical or criminal activity to thrive.

In law, it is considered that an employee has a duty to respect the confidentiality of the firm they work for as part of their terms of employment. The employee has privileged access to information and, from one perspective, it is this privileged access that the whistle blower abuses when the decision is made to expose bad practice. In healthcare settings it could be argued that breaching the confidentiality of the workplace means that the operating department worker was in breach of one of the main tenets of the Hippocratic oath (PBS, 2008): 'All that may come to my knowledge in the exercise of my profession or in daily commerce with men, which ought not to be spread abroad, I will keep secret and will never reveal'.

How then might one justify this breach of trust? To begin with, it is not entirely clear that the duty of confidentiality that is owed to an ordinary employer is the same as the duty owed to a hospital's operating department. Breaches of commercial confidentiality might lead to a loss of income for a business. However, preventing harm to the potential victims of malpractice in healthcare, and particularly in surgery, might lead to the conclusion that there were higher duties at stake than respecting Trust confidentiality. The public rightly regards as deeply reprehensible the practice of health workers covering up for each other's malpractice (Firtko & Jackson 2005).

There are, however, aspects of breaching confidentiality that are more difficult to deal with. It might be the case that the subject of the whistle blowing can only be revealed by revealing details of recognizable patients. These patients may not take the same view of the situation or they might agree with the stance but wish to be kept out of the glare of publicity. The Trust at the centre of Graham Pink's whistle blowing activities argued that their disciplinary action against Pink was not for revealing events in the Trust but rather for revealing information about patients. This information involved elderly and sometimes incontinent patients. Their relatives found reading details of their cases in the newspaper distressing and they complained.

Even where patient's details are not involved, there might still be difficulties. At the heart of a whistle blowing event is an accusation that things are not as they should be because of the actions of this or that person. The act of whistle blowing means that someone has to answer a charge. Accusing a practitioner of an improper practice can, in itself, be very damaging whatever the outcome of any subsequent enquiries. It seems harsh in the extreme for the practitioner's peers and possibly the general public to judge the practitioner as a result of an accusation made in public with no regard for the 'innocent until proven guilty' assumption.

These difficulties are recognized in professional codes and in law. A person is allowed to breach confidentiality where there is a reasonable public interest at stake. Employers may not discipline an employee who has breached confidentiality if the employee can demonstrate that there is a public interest in revealing the information. The Nursing and Midwifery Council (2008) Code of Conduct lists public interest as one of the reasons a nurse may disclose otherwise confidential information. The sting in the tail of this protection, however, is that the practitioner has to demonstrate that there is indeed a significant matter of public interest at play. What one person might regard as a scandalous situation might be regarded by another as relatively trivial.

In 1998, protection was offered in law for the whistle blower. In essence, this protection defined situations in which the whistle blower could justify the breach in the duty of confidentiality he or she owed to their employer. Only the disclosures defined in the Public Interest Disclosure Act of 1998 qualify for protection. These include 'any disclosure of information which, in the reasonable belief of the worker who makes the disclosure, tends to show that':

- a criminal offence has been committed, is being committed or is likely to be committed
- a legal obligation has not been complied with, is not being complied with or is likely not to be complied with
- a miscarriage of justice has taken place, is taking place or is likely to take place
- a risk to the health and safety of any individual has taken place, is taking place or is likely to take place
- damage to the environment has occurred, is occurring or is likely to occur
- deliberate concealment of information has occurred, is occurring or is likely to occur.

One of the effects of this legislation was to render void the so-called 'gagging clauses' that required workers to remain silent about what they observed at work as a matter of formal contractual agreement. Interestingly, however, the Public Interest Disclosure Act does not apply to situations that are also covered by the Official Secrets Act. Under its terms, no protection would be offered to, say, an operating department practitioner who reported poor conditions in operating departments in the armed forces (Hobby 2001).

Does whistle blowing, by definition, involve acceptance of a degree of personal risk?

Northumberland in Shakespeare's *Henry IV, Part II* says

> Yet the first bringer of unwelcome news
> Hath but a losing office, and his tongue
> Sounds ever after as a sullen bell,
> Remember'd tolling a departing friend.

Reporting on one's colleagues is never easy (Savill 2008). For many whistle blowers, serious repercussions follow their decision to 'go public'. In fairness, there are other circumstances in which the whistle blower speaks the mind of the rest of the workforce. Their act of standing up to be counted receives the support and the approval of their colleagues. The unpleasantness of their task is balanced by secondary benefits of popularity among long-suffering work colleagues. In addition, there might be widespread public support for the stance. Older readers may recall the fate of Clive Ponting, who reported to an MP the 'ministerial deception over the sinking of the Argentinean ship the *General Belgrano*' (McColgan 2000). In the court case which followed, Mr Ponting did not deny the facts offered by the prosecution but argued that he had a higher duty than that he owed to the legislation which was being used to prosecute him. So firm was his popular support that the jury failed to convict Mr Ponting, against the advice of the trial judge.

This question of support for one's actions in whistle blowing in itself raises some interesting ethical questions.

- If a person has chosen the press as the route by which to expose an unsatisfactory state of affairs, does the fact that he or she is paid for information alter their status as a whistle blower?

- Does the act of whistle blowing require that the act be selfless and without regard for any financial inducement?
- Does taking payment alter the moral value of what the whistle blower is attempting to achieve?
- Can it be argued that the act of informing on colleagues is so intrinsically stressful that some compensation for such courage is not only justifiable but well merited?

That the act of whistle blowing can be stressful is open to little doubt and it frequently carries enormous personal cost. The Public Interest Disclosure Act might protect whistle blowers from dismissal for whistle blowing under carefully defined circumstances but it cannot protect whistle blowers from the glares and the whispers of the colleagues who they have exposed. Operating departments are often closed and inward-looking environments where such behaviour, though well short of anything that could be defined as bullying or harassment, might make a person wish to leave their post. The Act will have little force in ensuring that, as a known whistle blower, the practitioner will have any success in finding another job. Neither will it compensate whistle blowers for any nervous exhaustion that the act of publicizing concerns might bring in its wake.

The first person in the UK to receive protection under the Public Interest Disclosure Act was a nurse who was sacked for reporting poor standards of care in a nursing home. His dismissal was deemed unfair and he received £23 000 in compensation. This is how he reported his subsequent experiences to the *Guardian* in 2000:

> It's been horrendous . . . the most difficult things to deal with were the isolation by other staff and being made to look like some ogre who had challenged the system . . . Good staff, staff who have a conscience, leave rather than blow the whistle.

In this case, there was clearly malpractice, which required rectification. However, in general, the practice of whistle blowing in the NHS might not always have such a benign aspect. On occasion, it might be possible to understand the perspective of someone who met the whistle blower with glares and whispers. Everyone is aware of situations in the NHS that are not ideal: surgical lists go on and on, operations are cancelled and members of staff are put under seemingly intolerable stress. Somehow the system survives, often depending on the dedication and the hard work of the staff.

In these situations, it seems very unjust that someone should expose the members of staff who are already under pressure to public humiliation and scorn. Leaving a service and exposing its faults to the public has the effect of burdening former colleagues with extra problems: continuing to run the service and dealing with the fallout from the whistle blowing. Looked at in this way, whistle blowing becomes a way of saving the conscience of the whistle blower at the expense of hard-working colleagues.

The manager of a whistle blower

The policies and procedures that Trusts rely on to determine the response to whistle blowing will derive in the main from the Public Interest Disclosure Act 1998. Most Trusts will have policies to ensure that allegations are noted, that these allegations are acted upon and that the person who is the subject of the allegation is made aware that a case has been made against them.

However, there may be occasions in which the member of staff making the allegations is not satisfied with the results of the investigation and goes outside the structures of the official procedure and, say, writes a letter to the local newspaper.

Procedure may dictate that the line manager takes part in the punishment of the individual concerned but, depending on the nature of the event, this might provoke some serious moral disquiet. This will especially be the case where the manager sympathizes with the staff member involved. In such circumstances, the decision that the manager will be called upon to make is which virtue he or she values most of all: loyalty to the organization or loyalty to a staff member who is under threat.

Even where the employee has gone through the official channels, there may be a moral duty on the manager to step in to defend the whistle blower from the hostility of fellow staff members, who may have been accused of poor standards of care. The recognition, on the one hand, that the role of the whistle blower is fraught with difficulty might incline a manager to the view that such a selfless act deserves protection and encouragement. On the other hand, it might seem that such an act has breached the trust that is essential between all members of an operating department staff beyond all repair and that in the interests of all concerned it might be best if the person at the centre of the publicity moved on. The approach to this issue is for the manager to make a decision and this will be part of the management style that the manager adopts. Similarly, the outcome is also for the manager to bear.

What about the subjects of whistle blowing?

So far this discussion has focused on the stress of making a whistle blowing allegation. However, for every allegation that is made there is a person or persons who are having an allegation made against them. The cost to the accused of such an allegation is rarely counted in the equation, yet this cost can be severe.

To count as an act of whistle blowing, as a subject worthy of going public, it might be considered that the accusation should be reasonably serious. For example, it would be hard to imagine an act of whistle blowing where the accusation was that, on occasions, the temperature in the operating department was a little high.

Being accused in an act of whistle blowing could have serious repercussions for an individual, even where investigation clears them of wrong doing. When accusations have been made, many professionals are all too prepared to believe the accusation on the grounds that there is 'no smoke without fire'. This could do irreparable damage to a practitioner's professional reputation even where subsequent investigation exonerates the accused. A notable exception to this is when a profession demonstrates a degree of professional solidarity, which amounts to an 'old boy network'.

There is every possibility that the accused will be suspended from his or her work pending an investigation of allegations, or at least that their records are seized for examination.

If the accusation is serious enough, there may well be lurid press coverage of accusations, with little or no coverage of any subsequent exoneration. This could have an enormous effect on the accused and on their family.

In these situations, it would be useful to the accused if one could rely upon the full support of the Trust management team. However, one of the first lessons that one might learn in the process is that the interests of the accused are not entirely identical to the interest of the Trust. The Trust's interests might be in preventing further damaging publicity and resolving the situation as soon as possible. A small compromise to the quality of someone's professional reputation might be considered a worthwhile price to pay to resolve an unhappy incident. The accused person might take an entirely different view of the nature of this compromise.

In such a situation, an accused person may wish to exercise caution before signing documents that accept blame for a situation that is the subject of the whistle blowing and to insist on representation at any formal investigation.

Conclusions

The act of whistle blowing is one that is fraught with difficulties, whether for the whistle blower or the accused. This action challenges important notions of trust and confidentiality at work. It also emphasizes to the highest degree the personal nature of commitment to patients and readiness to face the consequences if a situation becomes intolerable.

Although legal steps have been put in place to protect the whistle blower, it is hard to avoid the conclusion that this will always be an activity which carries personal consequences of the most radical kind.

REFERENCES

Firtko, A. & Jackson, B. (2005). Do the ends justify the means? Nursing and the dilemma of whistle blowing. *Australian Journal of Advanced Nursing,* **23**, 51–56.

Freedom to Care (2008). *Charge Nurse Graham Pink Blows Whistle on Nursing Understaffing.* http://www.freedomtocare.org/page73.htm (accessed 11 October 2008).

Hartley Brewer, J. (2000). Climate of fear let surgeon maim women. *The Guardian,* 2 June.

Hobby, C. (2001). *Whistleblowing and the Public Interest Disclosure Act 1998.* London: Institute of Employment Rights.

McColgin, A. (2000). Article 10 and the right to freedom of expression: workers ungagged. In Ewing KD (ed.) *Human Rights at Work.* London: Institute of Employment Rights.

Nursing and Midwifery Council (2008). *The Code. Standards of Conduct, Performance and Ethics for Nurses and Midwives.* London: Nursing and Midwifery Council.

PBS (2008). *The Hippocratic Oath.* http://www.pbs.org/wgbh/nova/doctors/oath_classical.html (accessed 11 October 2008).

Savill, R. (2008). Whistleblower nurse charged over Channel 4 Dispatches programme. *Daily Telegraph,* 24 June.

Shah, F. (2005). Whistleblowing: its time to overcome the negative image. *British Journal of Community Nursing.* **10**, 277–279.

18

A manager's experience of recruitment and retention

Jill Mackeen

Key Learning Points

- Understand the role of a manager in staff recruitment
- Identify the tasks involved with developing a recruitment strategy
- Understand interviewing of candidates
- Understand introducing new staff to the department
- Appreciate how to improve staff retention

The author was an operating department manager for many years and the chapter discusses some of the factors that this author found to be important while working in this position. Recruitment and retention is becoming increasingly important as the number of school leavers falls and the challenges for the NHS to increase its effectiveness and efficiency rise ever higher. Furthermore, many experienced managers left the NHS following service cutbacks that occurred in the first years of the twenty-first century. This chapter, therefore, offers a manager's eye view of the issues surrounding recruitment, interviewing, selection and retention of staff and how these can be addressed.

The modern operating theatre if it is to function properly relies on the manager to facilitate the needs of its staff, in terms of theatre personnel, equipment, appropriate training and a safe working environment. This chapter will concentrate on the human resource element, discussing the principles and management of staff recruitment, staff retention and sickness absence.

Prior to the start of a new financial year, a manager will need to assess the theatre's workforce strategy for the coming year. This is achieved by ascertaining who is currently in post, what vacancies exist and what staff numbers and skill mix is required to achieve the theatre's goals (Department of Health 2004).

The manager will need to assess the number of operating sessions that are to be staffed during the week. This may include elective day sessions, day theatre, trauma theatre, maternity or emergency theatre; the list is endless depending on the type of hospital theatre suite that is being managed. Each theatre will have different requirements depending on the type of surgery performed. The manager may have to accommodate some specialist operations where multiple surgical teams will be operating simultaneously.

When all this information has been gathered, the manager needs to assess if there is sufficient money within the budget to staff the theatre to the level of service required. It is at this time that the manager and finance department meet to discuss the funded staffing establishment. If there is insufficient money in the staffing budget, then the manager would need to put forward a 'case of need' to request further funding to overcome the deficit. This request will require accurate data to support the claim for additional funding. The theatre

Core Topics in Operating Department Practice: Leadership and Management, ed. Brian Smith, Paul Rawling, Paul Wicker and Chris Jones. Published by Cambridge University Press. © Cambridge University Press 2010.

information system may provide essential data in conjunction with senior staff, who can identify if there will be a change in the service provided from the previous year, for example additional operating lists, overrunning sessions or specific service initiatives. It would also be pertinent to include an assessment of the rules relating to the European Working Time Directive, as this may necessitate additional staff to comply with the rules in the future (Department of Health 2007a).

When this has been completed, the manager will need to look at the personnel currently in post and, where possible, predict if there is likely to be any changes to their personal situation in the next year. The manager may already know the people who will be retiring, but not those requesting part-time hours following a change in family or life circumstances. This is where the manager needs to review the staffing position on a regular basis and be approachable so that staff members may confide in the manager if a request for changes may be imminent.

If it is decided that additional staff need to be recruited, it is important that the manager reviews each vacancy and then decides how best to recruit to that vacancy. For example, is someone of the same grade needed or would it be better to recruit junior or part-time staff? There may be many variables that would give more flexibility within the staffing rosters. It should also be remembered that if a senior member of staff leaves the whole of their funding may not be replaced. The budget is based in many instances on the assumption that someone at a more junior level will be recruited into this position; consequently, the available funds may be reduced and this situation would need to be discussed with the finance team. Once finances have been agreed, then it is time to advertise.

It usually depends on the seniority of the position whether the manager decides to advertise locally or nationally. It can be very expensive to advertise in a professional journal but it may be necessary if it is important to attract the most suitable candidate. Advertising nationally may also be delayed by the frequency of publication; this is why it is important

that the manager is aware of the availability of professionals working within other hospitals locally (Mullins 1999).

The hospital website is a good place to advertise and it allows the prospective candidate to look at what can be gained from working within the organization. For potential candidates looking to move to a new area, general information of the location can also be included on the website, not just specific information relating to the position. In effect, it may be prudent to sell the area along with the specific hospital Trust.

When the human resources department begin the advertising process, they will need an up-to-date job description and personnel specification. The job description should detail what role the successful candidate would be expected to perform. This would include level and areas of responsibility, who would be their direct manager and what additional assistance they may need to progress within the role.

The personnel specification would include all the relevant requirements that the candidate must have, for example qualifications, current registration, previous experience, the ability to perform the role regarding shift patterns and on-call duties if required within the role. This information is important as the candidate can then assess if they are eligible to apply for the position and cannot state that they did not understand their commitment to the role. Accurate information at the outset can save time and expense for all concerned.

The advertisement should also include information on the application process and who they should contact for further information or to request an informal visit. The informal visit is another way of gleaning information both for the prospective candidate and the future employer. The information given to the prospective candidate should relate to the position and not specific questions that they are likely to be asked at interview.

If specific help regarding interview technique is required, then a person not on the interview panel could be made available for this purpose. The informal visit should also be encouraged for personnel applying internally. People currently working in the theatre department often believe that they know how the previous staff member performed the role and, therefore, what is required in this new position. This can be a false perception as the manager's idea of the new role may differ and the staff member should be encouraged to meet with the manager and discuss their ideas for the role. The internal candidate should also be reminded that they have to promote themselves at the interview and not rely on the fact that the panel have prior knowledge of the candidate. Many candidates have failed because they believe that the position is already theirs, but if the panel are going to be fair to all applicants they must judge on how they perform on the day.

Once the job has been advertised, candidates must apply for an application form or it may be possible to apply online. The application form must be completed and returned by a predetermined closing date. Application forms should not be accepted after this date unless previously agreed by the interviewing manager. On receipt, the human resources department will collect the application forms and forward these to the manager for scrutiny and a decision as to who should be called for interview.

The manager should meet with the other members of the interview panel and short list the suitable candidates with reference to the job description and person specification. The selection process is recorded by the panel, stating who was successful in being called for interview and who was rejected (NHS Employers 2008).

The candidates that have been rejected are sent a letter stating that they have not been successful on this occasion, sometimes offering a reason why, for example length of experience or less suitable than other candidates. The successful candidates are also informed by letter and given information as to the time and venue for their interview and what certificates and personal information they are required to provide at this time.

If candidates are to be tested, this should also be stated in the notification letter. Many interviews now expect the candidate to give a presentation on a stated topic. It is important that it is clearly stated what audiovisual aids will be available and to ensure that the equipment is in good working order on the day. It is also important that a member of the panel is able to help the candidate to set up their presentation if required. All information technology systems have their own individual gremlins!

At the same time as the human resources department send out the letters to the candidate's inviting them to attend for interview, references will be applied for unless the candidate specifically requests that the employing hospital do not request this information until they are likely to offer them the position. The candidate should be given approximately 10–14 days notice before attending for interview, especially if they are to prepare a presentation and arrange for time off from their current position. If staff members internally to the employing Trust are short listed then they should all be given the same time off prior to interview. This will ensure fairness to all, and if one candidate fails they will not be able to claim that they have been treated unfairly.

The timing of the interviews should be sufficient to allow for presentations, interview, candidate questions and then discussion among the interview panel members and completion of any documentation prior to moving on to the next candidate. If this is done properly, it will mean that candidates do not have too long to wait, which can exacerbate their nervousness. If there are multiple candidates, breaks need to be included for panel members to have a drink or lunch. This will ensure that every candidate is given the panel's full attention. It can be demanding for the interview panel when a significant number of candidates may be presenting for interview.

The members of the interview panel should be a senior grade to the position that is being considered at that time. At least one member of the interview panel should have been trained in interview techniques; usually this is in-house training by a senior member of the personnel department. This may vary between human resources departments, but usually a member of the human resources department will only be in attendance at interviews for positions at senior levels.

Prior to the day of interview, the panel should have met to consider what questions would be suitable to ask the candidates. The questions should be the same in fairness to all candidates but open to any questions relating to their particular application form. Questions should not be asked relating to gender, for example 'Will you be having children in the next five years?' 'How will you arrange child care?' The fact that they have applied means they should have considered personal issues, but you may wish to inform them that on-call duty will almost certainly be expected of them. The theatre candidate usually understands that this is likely to happen and often offer an explanation that they have already considered this or are used to being on-call, especially if applying for non-basic grade positions.

On the day of interview, it is important that the interview panel are relieved of all other duties for the duration of the interviews. Bleeps and telephones should be switched off out of respect for the candidates and to allow the panel to concentrate on the job in hand. The room used for interview should be quiet and suitable for the purpose.

At the start of the interview, it is normal for the chairperson to try and relax the candidate by getting them to talk about their journey or themselves before delving straight into questions. The pay scale, holiday entitlement, on-call arrangements and pension scheme are usually stated so that the candidate is fully aware of the position they are applying for and no misunderstanding will occur at a later date. If the candidate is required to deliver a presentation, this usually is next. The candidate will have prepared what they are going to deliver and this can also calm the situation as they should be confident in what they are presenting. The presentation should be relevant to the position and not try to trick the candidate; it allows them to demonstrate their depth of knowledge, experience and their ability to research information. The panel will be able to ask follow-up questions relating to the presentation.

Once this stage of the interview has been completed, the candidate needs to be given time to relax and each panel member will ask their questions. It is important how the questions are phrased, as this will determine the depth of the response by the candidate. This is also why it is important to spend time preparing the questions as an interviewing panel. An ambiguous or poorly phrased question will not aid the panel in deciding the most suitable candidate to fill the vacancy.

If the candidate is unable to answer a particular question, it can be rephrased but it is best not to linger too long over the topic as this may cause additional stress and completely ruin the candidate's chance of progressing further. The question may be returned to at the end of the interview if it is that important.

When the panel have completed their questions, it is time for the candidate to be given the opportunity ask questions. These questions often take the form of 'When will I start if successful?' 'Will there be an induction programme?' 'Will I be considered for attending courses?' These questions should be answered honestly as the candidate may be offered the position but if they do not feel welcome they may decline the offer and the panel is back to square one.

When the interview is completed, it is customary to thank the candidate for attending and inform them when and how they will hear the outcome of the interview. They should also be reminded that any offer of a position is subject to a satisfactory Criminal Records Bureau (CRB) check, references from two suitable referees and passing a medical examination (NHS Employers 2008).

On completion of the interviews, the panel members need to decide who they will appoint to the position. The information gained after each interview is then reviewed and only once a decision is made will the references be read. The references are used as a tool for confirming the decision already made and not for making the decision. In recent years, managers have been advised to limit the information given on references to confirm sickness absence and length of service. This prevents candidates who are not appointed from claiming that it was because of their poor references.

The successful candidate is usually contacted as previously stated and the position is offered, subject to the satisfactory CRB and medical examination. Once these details are available, a starting salary (based on previous earnings and experience) and commencement date is agreed by letter. The candidate will be asked to confirm in writing that they accept the position and it is usually at this time that the candidate will submit their resignation to their previous employer. If the panel do not feel that any candidate has the required attributes, then they should not appoint to the position but look at other options. It may be possible to transfer an existing member of staff to cover the vacancy until a suitable replacement is recruited at a later date (NHS Employers 2008).

If it is decided to recruit staff from overseas, it is important to get advice from the human resources department as it will require extra consideration; the candidate may need work permits, visas, confirmation as to qualifications, as well as a delay in obtaining references, CRB and medical examination. Interviews may be conducted using video conferencing. Overseas staff may also require additional training once in the UK to allow them to gain registration for practise in a qualified position (Department of Health 2007b).

Once the successful candidate has agreed to take the position, the manager needs to prepare for the arrival of the new employee and plan for an induction programme. This includes the new staff member meeting with personnel in human resources to sign a contract and being introduced to key staff within the theatre suite. All health and safety policies and relevant training will be arranged and undertaken to make the new employee eligible to work within the department.

It is also pertinent at this time that the new member of staff is informed about staff policies relating to duty rotas, annual leave, sickness absence and completion and submission of expense claim forms.

All new members of staff will feel vulnerable over the first few weeks, so every effort must be made by all staff to welcome the new arrival. Nominating a mentor can aid the settling-in period (Department of Health 2007c).

Staff retention

New and existing staff are all valuable to an organization; it has taken time and money to recruit and train them for their current position, so how they are dealt with on a daily basis can greatly enhance staff retention. Experienced theatre staff are greatly sought after, and if an individual does not feel appreciated then he or she is liable to leave and move to a neighbouring hospital.

Theatre managers do not have the ability to pay staff bonuses for good work, unlike some industries, but good communication and recognition of a job well done can improve morale; this is why team meetings with representatives of all staff grades can be beneficial. The theatre team relies on all its members to care for the patient and without this team commitment the theatre services will fail (Department of Health 2003a).

The retention of staff is paramount if the theatre is to achieve its target as set out in *The NHS Plan*. The manager needs to be aware that staff may need to work differently in order to achieve the correct work–life balance and should try to accommodate staff wishes if at all possible (Department of Health 2004).

Staff members now know that managers will have to take cognisance of requests in relation to the *Improving Working Lives* document (Department of Health 2003b). Hospitals cannot allow experienced staff to leave their position without trying to accommodate their request to improve their work–life balance.

Some managers offer school term-time contracts, reduction from full to part-time hours, job share and evening shifts as all these help to cover the needs of the theatres. When discussing requests for altered working times, the manager and the staff member have to understand that whatever is agreed the service to the patient must not be compromised. The manager also has to assess what shifts people already perform, and while it is important to consider if agreeing to a request will ensure that the member of staff stays in the employment, it is also important to ensure that this is not to the detriment of other staff members.

The manager may also agree to try a change in working arrangements for a limited period. This may give the employee time to look at other arrangements for childcare, for example, and the manager can see if these arrangements are sustainable.

The *NHS Child Care Strategy* (Department of Health 2007d) has been introduced by the government to try and provide more on-site child care facilities. It is hoped that this will prevent healthcare staff from leaving the NHS because they are unable to find child care that provides suitable cover for staff working a changing shift pattern.

Conclusions

It is clearly vital for a theatre manager to understand the process of recruitment and, more importantly, to understand why staff who are difficult to find and recruit need to be valued. A manager who understands these issues will be more likely to provide the benefits of a stable workforce capable of providing the highest quality care for patients.

REFERENCES

Department of Health (2003a). *Staff Involvement and Partnerships.* London: The Stationery Office; http://www.dh.gov.uk/en/Managingyourorganisation (accessed 1 September 2008).

Department of Health (2003b). *Improving Working Lives.* London: The Stationery Office; http://www.dh.gov.uk/en/Managingyourorganisation (accessed 1 September 2008).

Department of Health (2004). *Delivering Human Resources in the NHS Plan.* London: The Stationery Office; http://www.dh.gov.uk/en/publications (accessed 1 September 2008).

Department of Health (2007a). *European Working Time Directive.* London: The Stationery Office; http://www.dh.gov.uk/en/Managingyourorganisation (accessed 28 August 2008.

Department of Health (2007b). *International Recruitment: NHS Employers.* London: The Stationery Office; http://www.dh.gov.uk/en/Managingyourorganisation (accessed 28 August 2008).

Department of Health (2007c). *Human Resources and Training.* London: The Stationery Office; http://www.dh.gov.uk/en/Managingyourorganisation (accessed 28 August 2008).

Department of Health (2007d). *NHS Childcare Strategy.* London: The Stationery Office; http://www.dh.gov.uk/en/Managingyourorganisation (accessed 28 August 2008).

Mullins, L. J. (1999). *Management and Organisational Behaviour,* 5th edn. London: Prentice Hall.

NHS Employers (2008). *NHS Employment Check Standards.* Leeds: NHS Employers; http://www.nhsemployers.org/primary (accessed 28 August 2008).

FURTHER READING

Department of Health (2004). *Sickness Statistics.* London: The Stationery Office; http://www.dh.gov.uk/en/publications (accessed 28 August 2008).

Department of Health (2007). *National Recruitment Campaign.* London: The Stationery Office; http://www.dh.gov.uk/en/Managingyourorganisation (accessed 28 August 2008).

Department of Health (2007). *Work Related Stress Policies.* London: The Stationery Office; http://www.dh.gov.uk/en/Managingyourorganisation (accessed 28 August 2008).

19

The management of change

Paul Wicker

Key Learning Points

- Understand models of change that describe the stages or phases required to implement change
- Appreciate the tools and methods available to help in making changes
- Understand the basic steps in planning, organizing and executing a change management project

Introduction

Charles Handy is one of Britain's most prolific writers on the management of change. Handy's vision in 1976 was that organizations were set to change at an unprecedented rate (Handy 1993). History has supported this view and, consequently, 'effective management' and the 'management of change' can be seen as virtually synonymous.

The simplest way to make a change is sometimes just to do it. Sometimes, people will just say 'Great idea, lets get on with it then!' However, intuition alone may not always be enough, and planning can help to ensure that change happens the most effective way for the results that are required.

Modern organizations have to learn to change quickly and often in order to survive, often downsizing or being forced to become more effective in the process (Handy 1989). The primary task for all healthcare managers is to improve the quality of services while working within tight financial constraints. Management is no longer about maintaining the status quo – it is much more about

stimulating change and encouraging innovation to make improvements (Burnes 2000).

Every change programme involves three stages: the current stage, the transition stage and the desirable future change. All three require managing and all three compete for resources. In the author's experience, bringing about change requires a vast range of competencies to carry out a wide range of tasks, including the following:

- being clear about the purpose of the organization and the roles of the workers (what people do)
- communicating effectively (email, minutes, agendas, meetings, notes)
- building a shared vision for the future (where the organization is now, where it wants to go)
- establishing control of the change (reviewing progress, directing actions)
- building in learning resources for the staff (lectures, learning packs, education programmes)
- motivating staff (rewarding good practice, reducing poor practice)
- providing leadership (telling people what to do, asking people what they want to do)
- creating harmony between the informal and formal cultures of the organization (understanding what 'goes on')
- planning to deliver a quality service to the patients (what is in it for patients?)
- identifying external influences that might help or hinder the change process (contacting the director of nursing, accountants, managers or lecturers).

Core Topics in Operating Department Practice: Leadership and Management, ed. Brian Smith, Paul Rawling, Paul Wicker and Chris Jones. Published by Cambridge University Press. © Cambridge University Press 2010.

Change is never clean and tidy. It always has supporters and detractors; it will be scuppered and championed. It is about bending and controlling as well as tolerating ambiguity and uncertainty. It is about having the confidence to succeed when it is impossible to know whether it is the right change or not.

Models of change

Every organization has a culture and making changes is often about working with, manipulating or influencing the culture to make the changes happen. For example, Handy (1989) identified four main types of culture: power, role, task and person. He suggests that the power culture is one where there is a single powerful figure who makes all the key decisions. The person culture is rare and features a diverse group of people where each person's contribution is equal; combined they contribute to the aims of the organization. A role culture is defined by its many policies and procedures, each worker being strictly governed by those higher in the hierarchy. An organization that uses the task culture is project orientated; autonomous thinking and teamwork are encouraged in order to 'get the job done'.

Drennan (1992:3) defines culture rather succinctly as 'how things are done around here'. There are many other definitions and perspectives on culture, indicating that organizations are complex entities that require change managers to implement changes in different ways. Therefore, one way to ensure that a change project is effective is for change managers to identify the culture they are working in and decide the best way to go about making the change. One way to do this is by using a model of change.

There are many different models of change and choosing which one to use is often down to the nature of the change itself, the personal preferences of the change manager, based on their own knowledge or experience, and the features of the environment, or culture, in which the change is going to take place. This section provides three models to help to explain the steps involved in managing a change.

An organic approach to change

The 'simply do it' approach only works in an organization that allows its workers freedom of thought and action, such as in Handy's (1989) person or task culture. Although hospitals in the NHS are probably more like power or role cultures, no doubt teams or departments exist where individuals are allowed to exercise more freedom of thought. Turrill (1986) captures the essence of such an organization with his organic model of change (Fig. 19.1). This model subscribes to the belief that an innovative organization has the purpose, vision and beliefs to build in change as a norm. It encourages individuals to 'experiment' with different ways of working, and it reacts strongly and quickly to events such as critical incidents, government white papers, committee reports or senior staff concerns. Out of these experiments and ice-breaking events come successes, small or large. For example, a theatre team might react strongly to an anaesthetic incident, assemble a team of people to investigate it and from there start a strategy for change. The strategy then develops into actions from which comes learning, and further changes to the strategy, until it results in lasting change.

This approach to change builds on the successes of a few people with perhaps unrelated needs. Major hurdles do not have to be jumped (which reduces resistance to change) and there will be implicit support from the shop floor – where the change was started. The success of this model, or rather the success of the change, depends on an organization where the culture is innovative, supportive and open to change.

The change equation

David Beckhard (1969) describes the change equation as a way of understanding the motives of an individual or group. This equation expects that

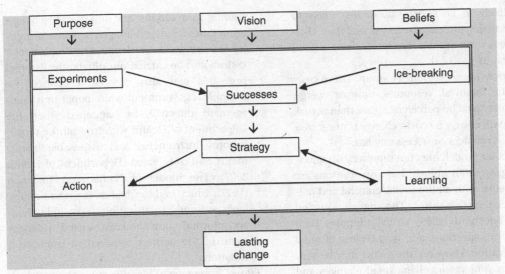

Figure 19.1 An Organic Model for Change. (Turrill 1986)

people will only make a change if there is something in it for them. Change is likely to happen only if the sum total of A, B and C is greater than D:

$$A + B + C > D$$

where A is the dissatisfaction of an individual or group with the current way of working, B is the vision of the individual or group for a better future, C is the existence of a safe and acceptable first step, and D is the cost to the individual or group.

It is the job of the change manager to assess or identify A, B and C, and to reduce the impact of D so the equation becomes true, as in the following examples.

The individual or group's dissatisfaction with the current way of working. People will not be motivated to change if they are comfortable with the current way of working. For example, for years practitioners wanted to retain swab racks in their operating rooms because they were comfortable with their use. It was only when information about the potential for infections such as the human immunodeficiency virus and hepatitis B became widely available that practitioners started to become uncomfortable with the practice. Using this model, a change manager would assess the level of comfort with the present system, and if people are comfortable for the wrong reasons then address the problem through a change project.

The individual's or group's vision for a better future. To sustain the change, the individual or group must share a vision for a better way of working. If the vision points to a worse way of working, then the change will not be sustained. For example, how many times has a manager seen members of their staff 'say' they are carrying out a change while in reality going on doing it the way they have always done it? A specific example is the use of cover gowns. While research has shown that cover gowns do get contaminated when used outside the operating department, and they are at best ineffective, their use persists because many practitioners prefer to slip on a cover gown rather than changing into 'outside' clothes. (Seavey 1996, Duquette-Peterson *et al.* 1999).

The existence of a safe and acceptable first step. The size of the first step, and the risks involved to the individual or group, may result in inertia. First steps are more acceptable if they are small and likely to be successful, or less likely to cause major embarrassment if they fail. Usually, less work and more reward is also a good motivator.

The costs to the individual or group. These costs may be financial, resources, time or energy. They may also be perceived rather than actual. There will always be costs: change is never free, nor is it painless or necessarily fair.

This particular model, may not suit every organization. Morgan (1986) argues that organizations are social systems, with all the social, cultural and political issues that this raises. The change equation model of Beckhard (1969) virtually ignores such aspects of organizations and is, therefore, limited in its application. However, the model may be very effective for projects involving small changes and managed within small teams, since it helps the change manager to identify very quickly the main reasons for the change, where the resistance to change will come from and gives an indication of how to start the change process.

Lewin's three-phase model

Kurt Lewin's model (1951) is much quoted in the literature (Green & Cameron 2004). Although it has come under various degrees of criticism over the years, it appears to fit well into the power or role culture of the NHS. Lewin identifies three phases in any change programme.

1. Unfreezing: giving people time to adjust to the idea of change. Recognizing their achievements and 'putting them to bed' to make room for new achievements.
2. Moving: putting the change into effect.
3. Refreezing: institutionalizing and consolidating new behaviours and establishing new norms. This requires consideration of new tasks, individuals and the formal and informal systems.

Phase 1: unfreezing. Unfreezing events are those which encourage a change to happen. Such events might include a patient injury, an adverse incident or a 'near miss'; the event itself will probably be unplanned and unexpected, leading to a sudden and unexpected change. Sometimes a senior manager, person in authority or committee can demand that a particular task should be carried out differently. External pressures can also enforce a change, for example a government white paper or a management directive, as happened when the Department of Health withdrew all the tonsillectomy instruments and disposable instruments had to be used (Department of Health 2007). The model of Nadler and Tushman (1977), which is described in the next section, looks at formal organization, tasks, individuals and informal culture and can be used to identify some of the actions required to unfreeze a situation.

Phase 2: moving. This phase is about taking actions to ensure the change happens. Bearing in mind the dangers of managing change, it makes sense to assume that careful planning should go into the implementation stage. The first rule has to be that 'things will go wrong' no matter how well a group or individual plans change. The effects of the change will cause new resistances to arise, unexpected events to occur and the change will not happen in the way the change manager expected. So, it is always necessary to monitor the change and take action as it is required. The tools in the next section provide techniques for managing this step of the change process.

Phase 3: refreezing. Refreezing captures the need to embed firmly in the organization what has been achieved in order to avoid successes from reverting to the 'old ways'. If unfreezing was about grieving for the old way, then refreezing is about celebrating the new way of working and recognizing and rewarding new behaviours.

Tools and methods of change

Lewin's model (Lewin's 1951, Green & Cameron 2004) is used to look at the various tasks that need to be carried out during unfreezing, moving and

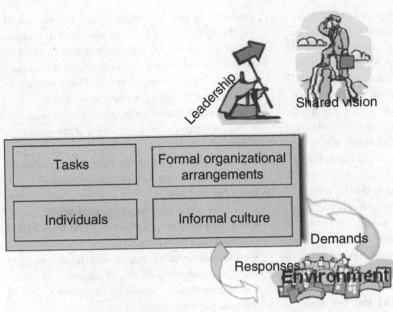

Figure 19.2 Diagnostic Tool. (Nadler and Tushman 1977)

refreezing phases, and the tools that are available to carry out these stages.

The unfreezing phase

Change managers can use diagnostic tools to examine the team, department or organization to ensure that their plan for change addresses the right problem.

The first step in managing the change should be to answer the questions 'What is the problem that requires you to make a change?' or 'What changes do I need to make my area work more effectively?' This section provides a way of looking at each of the separate parts of an organization and how they relate to one another, to help in understanding the current situation and what the change team needs to change.

Figure 19.2 is a diagnostic tool adapted from Nadler and Tushman (1977). The purpose of the tool is to try to clarify all the parts of the organization that which influence the change. These can be divided into the environment outside the organization, the internal organization and the shared vision.

The *environment* outside the organization imposes continual demands on the organization, which, in turn, must make suitable responses.

The *internal organization* can be divided into four areas: the formal organization, the tasks, the individuals and the informal culture.

Formal organization. This includes such characteristics as lines of accountability, information systems, control mechanisms, job definitions, policies and procedures and meetings. The policies, procedures and ways of working were designed for the old way and will continue to use resources until they are changed. The change manager must identify and address problems with outdated systems and paperwork.

Tasks. This includes looking at the nature of the jobs, the characteristics of the work, how the organization achieves the objectives and how it provides the service. The change manager must review jobs, roles and tasks that members of staff undertake. Do they still need doing? Can people work differently? What work will stop to let people do the new work?

Individuals. This includes the people who make the organization run: their skills, knowledge, qualities, qualifications, attitudes, beliefs and behaviour. In any team, there will be the innovators, who are good at dreaming up new ideas, conservators who are staunch supporters of the old ways and consolidators who are good at getting on with the work. The consolidators will be most important at this stage, while the innovators may prevent a new way of working from becoming established as they will always be looking for different ways to do the work.

Informal culture. This involves 'the way things are done', rites and rituals, power bases, allegiances, beliefs, norms and networks. The change manager must look at the wider environment, such as informing senior management, ensuring that patients understand the change, and ensuring that all the key stakeholders understand and agree with the changes. Addressing the informal organization and making the cultural changes can take the longest and be the hardest part of any change. This part is about changing the way 'we do things around here'.

The *shared vision* is the description of a better future. Finally, *leadership* encompasses the activities that keep the organization moving towards the shared vision.

These parts of the organization coexist: change one and the others change too. For example, if a task changes, individuals must change to accommodate the change (e.g. through further training). This may call for a change in the informal culture (shorter tea breaks) and a change in the formal structure (a change in a policy).

Consequently, when thinking about a change, the tool can help the change manager to understand the current situation and how it might respond to the changes. It can also be used to help to pinpoint areas that need attention to ensure that change happens. For example, the change manager might decide to use a particular individual's skills in a different part of the organization (because he or she is good at consolidating change but not instigating it).

The lists below are what might be generated using the tool (Nadler & Tushman 1977) to analyse a change project to introduce preoperative visiting:

- *formal organizational arrangements*, for example:
  - theatre management system has section to record outcomes of preoperative visit
  - job description includes preoperative visiting
  - preoperative policies include a section on preoperative visiting
  - preoperative visiting procedure included in operating department documentation
- *tasks*, for example,
  - time required for preoperative visiting
  - role description: practitioner must understand boundaries to the role
  - equipment required: none specifically required but depends on patient's condition
  - documentation: assessment sheet, record sheet, patients' notes
- individuals, for example:
  - Dr Jones is interested in the project
  - Dr Smith believes that patients do not require preoperative visiting by practitioners because anaesthetists do it anyway
  - the principal operating department practitioner (ODP) has never done preoperative visiting and does not understand its purpose
  - recovery staff currently undertake preoperative visiting but do not pass on information to operating department staff
- *informal culture*, for example:
  - team leaders in operating rooms organize roles and tasks for staff and may feel upstaged by the introduction of a new role
  - staff take early morning tea breaks before the list starts, when preoperative visiting might be undertaken
  - anaesthetists, in general, are not supportive because they worry that practitioners will tell the patient about their anaesthetic
  - surgeons on the whole do not care if it happens or not, unless it delays the start of their list
- *shared vision*, for example:
  - the staff in teams 1 and 2 are interested in this project but the staff in team 4 do not want to

know anything about it and team 6 may be interested but they want to wait and see what reception the project gets

- the current role description and policy were written 8 years previously
- the corporate mission statement supports the idea of preoperative visiting
- *leadership*, for example Joe Wright would be an ideal leader; there are also several interested practitioners in main theatres and in recovery.

The moving phase

The moving phase is one of the most important stages of the project because it is when most of the activity takes place, and it is a key stage for deciding whether the change will be a success.

There are many reasons why a project will go wrong, for example:

- lack of understanding of the need for the change (people may believe, for example, that 'glutaral-dehyde is safe if used properly')
- lack of skills and knowledge to implement the change ('I don't know how to do it that way')
- lack of resources ('procurement won't let us order that model')
- current organizational arrangements are incompatible with new methods of working ('there isn't enough time to do it that way')
- motivation to change is low (I can't see anything positive coming out of it').

The change manager must implement solutions for each of the identified problems. For example, participants can be kept informed through emails, letters, talks or lectures. There will no doubt be a need to provide training and education sessions and to ensure that the correct resources are available prior to introducing the change. It will also be necessary to update the institution's policies and procedures when introducing the change and to maintain motivation to change by undertaking regular observation and feedback with rewards and punishments.

To manage change effectively, the change manager has to address all the areas identified during the unfreezing stage and move them to the new position. The four *change tools* described here may help to clarify what has to be done to make the change work successfully. The four tools are:

- environmental mapping: identifying the key areas within the organization or area and how the change will impact on them
- commitment planning: identifying a critical mass of supporters and what has to be done
- force field analysis: forces for and against the change
- change equation: identifying why and how it has to be done.

Environmental mapping

Organizations are made up of increasingly complex parts. For example:

trauma team. . . is part of. . .
orthopaedic service. . . is part of. . .
critical care directorate. . . is part of. . .
surgical services. . . is part of. . .
St Elsewhere Hospital. . . is part of. . .
University Hospital NHS Trust. . . is part of. . .
NHS in Scotland. . . is part of. . .
NHS in UK. . . is part of. . .
World Health Organization. . . is part of. . .
and so on.

Each subsystem will have a part to play in achieving the objectives of the system that it serves. If such a contribution does not exist, then the subsystem serves no purpose and should be (or will be) removed.

None of the identified systems will be closed: each one interacts with the others in either a greater or lesser way and the successful management of these boundaries is a key feature of change management. For any particular change project, it is assumed that the area where the change is taking place is the 'system', and all the other systems make up the environment, which makes demands on the system. Think of the interaction between these systems in terms of *demands made* by the environment and *responses required* of the system. For example, Fig. 19.3 shows a simple environmental

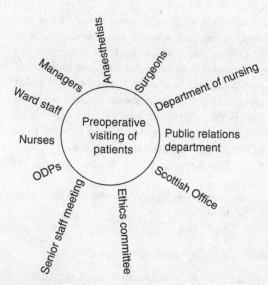

Figure 19.3 Simple representation of a Environmental Map for Preoperative visiting.

Table 19.1 An example of commitment planning

Key players	Not committed (Oppose)	Let	Help	Make
Nurse X				XO
Nurse Y and Z		X	O	
ODP A and B		X		O
Anaesthetist	X	O		
Surgeons		XO		
Ms X, Senior hospital manager	X	O		
Theatre manager		X		O

map to describe the preoperative visiting example. Once all the systems have been identified, the team may decide that some are irrelevant. One way to identify the critical systems is to say, 'What will happen if I ignore this system?' If the answer is nothing or very little, then it can safely be ignored; if not, then it is a key system.

Having identified the key systems, the change manager must examine the work that needs to be done. For example, anaesthetists are likely to be affected in some way by the implementation of a preoperative visiting service. Therefore, some of the following steps may help:

- coopt an anaesthetist on to the change group
- ensure that the anaesthetists know the purpose of the preoperative visiting role
- ensure that the practitioners know the purpose of the role
- confirm support for the role with the Royal College of Anaesthetists
- match the role to national standards, such as the Quality Assurance Agency, Health Professions Council, Nursing and Midwifery Council or professional bodies such as the Association for Perioperative Practice.

Identifying the key systems and considering all the aspects of the changes required helps the change manager to understand the work that needs to be done to complete the change process effectively.

Commitment planning

The aim of commitment planning is to help to build a critical mass of supporters who will help to make the change. The levels of commitment exhibited by individuals can be described as:

- not committed: likely to oppose the change
- let happen: will not oppose the change but will not actively support it
- help to happen: will support the change but only if someone else takes the lead
- Make happen: will lead the change and make it happen.

Each individual is rated with an 'X' to indicate their present position, and an 'O' to indicate the degree of commitment needed. In the example on preoperative visiting, this might be illustrated as in Table 19.1.

The difference between the X and the O points to the work required to make the project work. So, for example, nurse X is committed and will make the change happen. The nurses will let it happen, but that is not enough; they have to help it to happen otherwise the project will flounder. The ODPs need to be involved as well and must become active in the change. The anaesthetist does not like it; his or

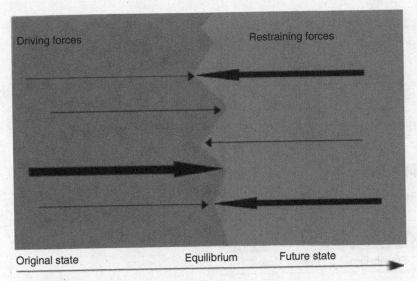

Figure 19.4 Diagram of a Force Field Analysis.

her active support is not required but he or she must let it happen.

Once the required level of commitment of individuals is identified, there are several ways of gaining it, usually based on interpersonal skills and using the systems to advantage. For example:

- use reward and punishment, for example increased status, or recognition of achievements
- change the systems of work, making it easier for the person to work with the change
- support people through education about the issues concerning them
- act as a role model, showing commitment and enthusiasm to the change
- use peer pressure to persuade the non-conformists to adopt the new ways
- encourage networking and allow people to use other people's successful ideas
- be prepared to negotiate and trade advantages and incentives.

Force field analysis

In the tool developed by Kurt Lewin (1951), the assumption is that there will always be two sets of forces in any change situation: one for and one against. The forces can be displayed on a chart to show their direction and relative strengths. The forces may be perceived or actual. For example, if members of staff believe that managers are going to make them redundant (although that may not be the object) then they will resist the change. The list of forces can be developed by brainstorming or by using a diagnostic model (e.g. that of Nadler and Tushman (1977)). Figure 19.4 shows the basic structure of the force field analysis. Sometimes it is useful to cluster the forces under subheadings, for example,

- *personal*: fear of redundancy, loss of pay, personal gain
- *interpersonal*: A does not talk to B; C does not support the change; D is a staunch supporter
- *intergroup*: nurses versus ODPs, practitioners versus surgeons, surgeons versus anaesthetists, ODPs versus managers
- *organizational*: shortage of resources, allocation of staff, policies
- *technological*: computerized records, equipment
- *environmental*: increasing numbers of patients, law, autonomy, registration.

After producing a chart, for example a force field chart for preoperative visiting (Fig. 19.5), the first

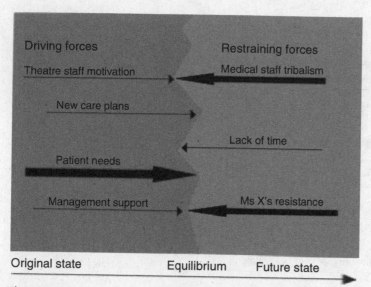

Figure 19.5 Example of a simple force field analysis for introducing preoperative visiting.

step is to think about reducing the restraining forces. Pushing the driving forces harder should be avoided as this will only increase the resistance.

A change manager, group or committee may decide that the change project is unachievable after considering all the factors involved. Taking that decision may save much time and effort. If it is achievable, the analysis will help the change manager to have a better idea about where to expend energies for the maximum effect.

The refreezing phase

The refreezing phase is essential in the management of change but is often forgotten because it lacks the excitement or energy of the other stages. If it is not utilized, behaviours may revert to the 'old way of doing things' or, even worse, people may say they are doing something when the reality is that they are not.

The information gained during the previous steps may be useful in this area too. For example, commitment planning may have identified individuals who will carry through and sustain the changes. These are the 'champions' and need to be nurtured

and encouraged. There will also be individuals who either ignore the changes or undermine them. They too need to be managed and their resistance either lowered or made ineffectual.

Bridges (1991) relates this stage to leadership techniques and offers various suggestions for marking the end of the old ways and the start of the new. For example, he supports good planning to ensure that managers understand who is likely to be affected by the change. Those who lose the most (e.g. job role, networks or status) will be the most likely to resist the change the most. Other actions can include:

- allowing people to discuss the effects of the change openly
- offering incentives for accepting the change, such as training, education, new roles or better working patterns
- finding a way to mark the end of the old ways, such as holding a launch of the new way
- remembering the old way with pride, as a necessary step towards the new and better way.

The leadership skills of the manager can do much to ensure that staff follow through the change as desired. The main techniques available for the manager to use during this phase are through developing new policies and procedures, and monitoring and review using audit techniques. Refreezing can, therefore, take a long time to achieve, and is a key step to whether the change is sustained.

Resistance to change

Change may need to be brought about without the aid of an unfreezing event, such as a patient incident or policy change. In these situations, there is likely to be resistance to change. Potential sources of resistance must be identified and decisions made on how to overcome them.

Kotter (1996) identified four reasons people resist change:

- self interest: a wish not to lose something
- a misunderstanding and mistrust of the change and its implications
- a belief that the change does not make sense to them or the organization
- a low tolerance for change.

Kegan & Lahey (2001) also believe that employees resist change because of a hidden agenda, known as a 'competing commitment'. When the hidden agenda is uncovered, the reason for the resistance to change becomes glaringly obvious. For example, practitioners may resist carrying out preoperative visiting if they miss an early morning coffee break or if it interrupts another important task.

To address these areas of resistance, and effectively unfreeze a situation, Kotter and Schlesinger (1979) suggest addressing the following areas. First, participants need to know about the change: why it is needed and what the advantages and disadvantages are. This ensures that people do not resist simply because they do not know about it. Telling people about the change ensures transparency and shows them that their opinion is respected and their needs are respected, as well as helping to manage the change effectively. Participants also need to be involved in the change, for example by asking their opinions and acting on their ideas. This draws people into the change and enlists their help. They may become staunch supporters of the change, defending it when the change team are not there to do it themselves. Participants will need support during the difficult period of change, for example through time for education or giving leeway on policy implementation until the timing is suitable.

The change manager will need to negotiate and agree changes with the people being affected. For example, an incentive for change in one area could include reducing workload in other areas.

Including those people who will resist the change can be a good tactic to allow them to see both sides of the need for change and to be able to influence the way it is implemented. For example, coopting anaesthetists or surgeons into a project group looking at implementing preoperative visiting can mean that their agendas are also addressed and professional boundaries are crossed with support on either side. Where speed of change is essential, coercion may be required and managers may have to compel employees to make the change, through enforcing policy changes for example. This is a dangerous tactic that can encourage high resistance to change if the change is an unpopular one.

While addressing resistance to change is an important part of change management, it is vital to understand that resistance is not always bad and may, in fact, be used constructively to implement the change. Piderit (2000) points out that some people may resist change because they think it is bad for the organization. Harnessing resistance of this kind may lead to the development of further alternatives or the introduction of more efficient changes, paradoxically helping the organisation to make changes which may be beneficial to it. Folger and Skarlicki (1999) claim that not all changes are appropriate and legitimate resistance may modify the change into something more effective for the organization.

Case study: planning and achieving a transfer of services to a new hospital

The purpose of this case study is to outline a possible strategy for managing a major change, in this example a move of services from one hospital to another. The author would like to thank Claire Campbell for permission to use the information contained within this case study, which is entirely fictitious.

Surviving as a manager of change requires many skills. For example, it would be sensible to assume that if managers are going to succeed, they will need to be empathic to their workers' needs and stay optimistic. Similarly, it would be more effective to ensure success in the early stages of the project by encouraging supporters rather than trying to overcome the resisters. Early experiments or pilot studies should be well resourced, with key people identified who will make the change happen, ensuring the project does not fall at the first hurdle.

The project will be described under the following headings:

- diagnosis: what needs to change
- planning
- organizing.

Diagnosis

Using Nadler and Tushman's (1977) diagnostic tool, the following areas were identified as being influenced by the change.

Phase 1 of the new St Elsewhere Hospital, due to open in 2009, will house elective and emergency theatres for ENT, gynaecology, obstetrics and elective orthopaedics. These are currently provided on four separate sites and work independently of one another. In phase one, gynaecology and obstetrics will share a suite, as will ENT and orthopaedics.

There are four groups of theatres, which are separated both geographically and by surgical specialty. Obstetric surgery is currently staffed by midwives, with theatre input for anaesthetic support only.

These four units will be transferred into the new structure. ENT and elective orthopaedics will share a suite of eight theatres and gynaecology and obstetrics a suite of five.

Planning

The key challenges presented in integrating and transferring these services were identified using the diagnostic tools and can be summed up as:

- education and training
- communication
- motivation, at all levels
- leadership: organizing the actions required
- staff support.

Education and training

Education and training strategies include a wide range of activities aimed at all those associated with the change process involved in integrating and transferring services.

Clinical staff will need education and training to deal with the change in surgical specialties undertaken in the theatres, and the recovery services will also need support to handle the change in structure. The use of teaching packages as well as 'hands on' experience will aid in implementing this change in practice. Support may be gained from others, for example the education coordinator and midwifery staff.

Education and training may provide support for members of staff holding posts that may require regrading, as individuals may wish to develop other clinical and managerial skills to apply for different posts within the new structure.

Identifying education and training opportunities for staff within the new structure may reduce resistance to the change process, for example extension and development of skills within new areas.

Communication

Communication is central to any strategy identified, as a failure in communication and information supplied will prevent successful implementation, regardless of the value of the strategy utilized. Communication strategies must allow two-way communication – from the top down and from the bottom up – and include all who are potentially affected by the change.

ID	Task Name	Duration	Start	Finish
1	PROJECT INITIATION	139 days?	Mon 02/01/08	Mon 14/07/08
2	Assemble project team	24 days	Mon 02/01/08	Mon 04/02/08
3	First Meeting	1 day	Mon 04/02/08	Mon 04/02/08
4	Develop main aims and objectives for team	0 days	Mon 04/02/08	Mon 04/02/08
5	Visit new premises	1.5 days	Mon 04/02/08	Wed 06/02/08
6	Liaise with architect	1 day	Wed 06/02/08	Wed 06/02/08
7	Inform surgeons and anaesthetists of changes to theatre routines	10 days	Thu 07/02/08	Wed 20/02/08
8	Meet with staff	21 days	Mon 17/03/08	Mon 14/04/08
9	Identify key learning deficits	23 days	Mon 14/04/08	Wed 14/05/08
10	Design schedule of learning	21 days	Fri 16/05/08	Fri 13/06/08
11	Produce Report for Board	116 days?	Mon 04/02/08	Mon 14/07/08
12	Board Approval	1 day	Mon 14/07/08	Mon 14/07/08
13	Untraining Activities	194 days?	Wed 16/07/08	Mon 13/04/09
14	Staff meeting to present Report and action plan	1 day?	Wed 16/07/08	Wed 16/07/08
15	Implement teaching package for new obs & Gynae staff	44 days	Wed 16/07/08	Mon 15/09/08
16	Implement teaching package for new ENT staff	44 days	Wed 16/07/08	Mon 15/09/08
17	Implement teaching package for new Orthopaedic staff	44 days?	Wed 16/07/08	Mon 15/09/08
18	Implement teaching package for team leaders	66 days	Wed 16/07/08	Wed 15/10/08
19	Staff meeting to present update of action plan	1 day?	Wed 15/10/08	Wed 15/10/08
20	Visits to new premises	67 days?	Wed 15/10/08	Thu 15/01/09
21	Staff meetings to review preparation	42 days?	Thu 15/01/09	Fri 13/03/09
22	Meetings with estates to check on resources	22 days?	Fri 13/03/09	Mon 13/04/09
23	SIGN OFF	1 day	Mon 13/04/09	Mon 13/04/09
25	Moving Activities	16 days	Fri 01/05/09	Mon 25/05/09
26	Transfer of services	0 days	Fri 01/05/09	Fri 01/05/09
27	a) Closure of operating theatres	5 days	Mon 04/05/09	Fri 08/05/09
28	b) Packing of equipment	5 days	Mon 04/05/09	Fri 08/05/09
29	c) Moving of equipment	2 days	Mon 11/05/09	Tue 12/05/09
30	d) Setting up new operating theatres	2.6 days	Wed 13/05/09	Fri 15/05/09
31	e) Testing of equipment	0 days	Tue 19/05/09	Tue 19/05/09
32	f) Staff meeting to identify problems	0 days	Wed 20/05/09	Wed 20/05/09
33	g) Staff training with new equipment	2 days	Thu 21/05/09	Fri 22/05/09
34	h) Start operating	0 days	Mon 25/05/09	Mon 25/05/09
35	SIGN OFF	0 days	Mon 25/05/09	Mon 25/05/09
37	Retraining activities	67 days?	Mon 01/06/09	Tue 01/09/09
38	Staff meeting to review moves and develop action plan	0 days	Mon 01/06/09	Mon 01/06/09
39	Assemble group to review policies and procedures	6 days	Mon 01/06/09	Mon 08/06/09
40	Rewrite policies and procedures	67 days	Mon 01/06/09	Tue 01/09/09
41	Review facilities problems	1 day	Wed 01/07/09	Wed 01/07/09
42	Staff meeting to review issues and develop action plan	1 day?	Wed 01/07/09	Wed 01/07/09
43	Set up new teaching programmes	23 days	Wed 01/07/09	Fri 31/07/09
44	SIGN OFF	45 days?	Mon 01/06/09	Fri 31/07/09
47	PROJECT COMPLETION	1 day?	Fri 03/07/09	Fri 03/07/09

Project: Change Project
Date: Sun 11/11/07

Task
Critical Task
Progress
Milestone
Summary
Rolled Up Task
Rolled Up Critical Task
Rolled Up Milestone
Rolled Up Progress
Split
External Tasks
Project Summary
Group By Summary
Critical Task

Page 1

Figure 19.6 Example of an action plan using Microsoft Project.

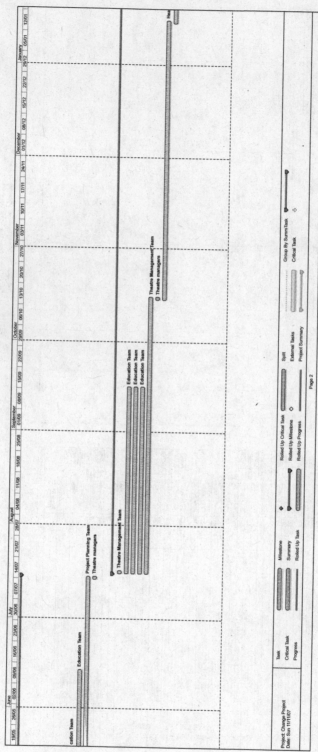

Figure 19.6 (cont.)

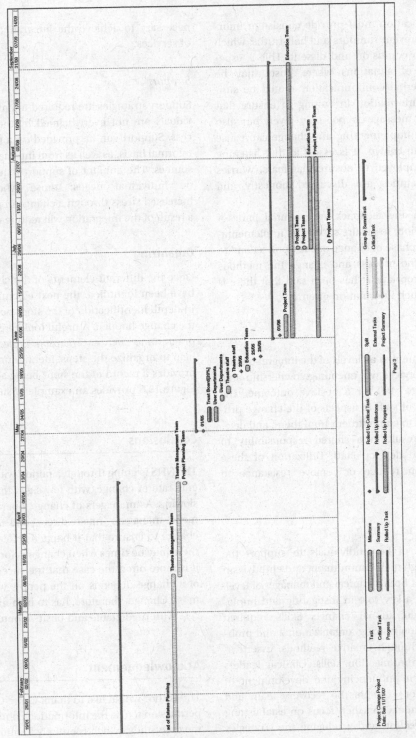

Figure 19.6 (cont.)

Communication must provide consistent information to prevent rumours and half-truths, which may lead to confusion and dissent. This is especially true of situations where posts may be regraded. Verbal communication should be supported by information in writing to ensure that the correct message is not only given but also received. As implementing any change can cause fear of the unknown, it is essential that listening skills are employed to ensure that fears, worries and uncertainties are discussed honestly and openly.

Evaluation and feedback are essential parts of communication, to ensure successful implementation of each phase of change or each project and to learn from the process and change the methods used, if appropriate. It has been said that there is rarely too much information given.

Motivation

Staff involvement at all levels of the integration and transfer of services will encourage ownership and, thus, motivate staff for a positive outcome. The participation of staff in aspects of the change process can lead to commitment from them, and delegation will result in a shared responsibility to empower and develop staff. Utilization of these strategies can reduce or remove resistance to change.

Leadership

Identification of key individuals to support the change through their commitment and enthusiasm is necessary at both a clinical and managerial level. Leaders have a key role in instigating and implementing organizational change. Skills required include decision making, organizational and problem solving through creative methods, assertiveness and communication skills. Clinical leaders are essential in influencing the development of new teams, for example the recovery team and managerial leaders can then focus on establishing the future direction and producing the strategies necessary to achieve the integration and transfer of services.

Support

Support strategies are required to ensure that individuals are not overwhelmed by the change process. Support can be provided on a formal and an informal basis, as well as from internal and external sources. The amount of support required depends on individual needs; those who experience increased stress through a change in post or role as a result of the integration will require more support.

Organizing

Once the different elements of the change process have been identified, the next essential step is the in-depth identification of the steps needed to make the change happen. A useful tool here is a software programme such as *Microsoft Project*, which can help to organize the steps, identify timescales, and provides a record of the steps being accomplished. Figure 19.6 provides an example of such a plan.

Conclusions

The NHS is going through a period with a phenomenal rate of change, with few signs that the rare is slowing. As managers of change, operating department managers must direct and control that change to ensure that it happens effectively. While there may be times when change is forced through, it is more often the case that the success or failure of a change depends on the people who it affects most. Change, therefore, has to be a managed process with predictable and positive outcomes.

Acknowledgement

The author would like to thank Claire Campbell for permission to use the information contained within the case study, which is entirely fictitious.

REFERENCES

Beckhard, R. (1969). *Organization Development: Strategies and Models*. Reading, MA: Addison-Wesley.

Bridges, W. (1991). *Managing Transitions: Making the Most of Change*. Reading, MA: Addison-Wesley.

Burnes, B. (2000). *Managing Change: A Strategic Approach To Organisational Dynamics*. Harlow, UK: Pearson.

Department of Health (2007). *Protecting the Public*. London: The Stationery Office; http://www.dh.gov.uk/en/Aboutus/MinistersandDepartmentLeaders/ChiefMedicalOfficer/Features/FeaturesBrowsableDocument/DH_5663255 (accessed 5 November 2007).

Drennan, D. (1992). *Transforming Company Culture*, p. 3. London: McGraw-Hill.

Duquette-Petersen, L., Francis, M.E., Dohnalek, L., Skinner, R. & Dudas, P. (1999). The role of protective clothing in infection prevention in patients undergoing autologous bone marrow transplantation. *Oncology Nursing Forum*, **26**, 1319–1324.

Folger, R. & Skarlicki, D.P. (1999). Unfairness and resistance to change: hardship as mistreatment. *Journal of Organizational Change Management*, **12**, 35–50.

Green, M. & Cameron, E. (2006). *Making Sense of Change Management*. London: Kogan Page.

Handy, C. (1989). *The Age of Unreason*. London: Arrow.

Handy, C. (1993). *Understanding Organisations*. London: Penguin.

Kegan, R. & Lahey, L. (2001). The real reason people won't change. *Harvard Business Review*, **79**, 85–89.

Kotter, J.P. (1996). *Leading Change*. Boston, MA: Harvard Business School Press.

Kotter, J.P. & Schlesinger, L.A. (1979). Choosing strategies for change. *Harvard Business Review*, **57**, 106.

Lewin, K. (1951). *Field Theory in Social Science: Selected Theoretical Papers* (Cartwright, D., ed.). New York: Harper.

Morgan, G. (1986). *Images of Organisations*. Beverley Hills, CA: Sage.

Nadler, D. & Tushman, M.L. (1977). *Perspectives of Behaviour*. London: McGraw-Hill.

Piderit, S.K. (2000). Rethinking resistance and recognizing ambivalence: a multidimensional view of attitudes toward an organizational change. *Academy of Management*, **794A**, 783.

Seavey, R.L. (1996). Eliminating cover gowns for perioperative personnel. *AORN Journal*, **63**, 465–466.

Turrill, T. (1986). *Change and Innovation: A Challenge for the NHS*. London: Institute of Health Services Management.

Index

Printed in the United States
By Bookmasters